HABIT LAUNCH

10-Step Formula to Tailor Routines You Love to Perform and Skyrocket Your Well-being

Gregor Moniuszko

Gregor Moniuszko
Walcownicza 36A
04-921 Warsaw
Poland
http://moniuszko.net

Written in 2016-2017 by Gregor Moniuszko

Edited by Amanda Larson

Book and Cover design by Gregor Moniuszko

ISBN: 9781973224129

First Edition: November 2017

10 9 8 7 6 5 4 3 2 1

Dedication

*This book is dedicated to everyone who is not afraid
of shifting the paradigm.*

GM

CONTENTS

Habit Launch Extras

Free PDF Workbook

Do exercises described in this book in a well-organized manner.

Bonus Material

Check out the bonus material for this book and get:

- Different points of views

- Extended information

- Additional examples

- And more

Get all the extras at:

http://moniuszko.net/habit-launch-extras/

What others have said about *Habit Launch*

There are lots of books on how to create and maintain a new habit. What makes this book unique is that it helps you figure out WHICH habit you should create.

Wendy Werneth, a.k.a The Nomadic Vegan, author of *Veggie Planet*

The most awesome book in the known universe about validating your habits . . . This book is like a Tesla car . . . The more you use it, the more you realize how much thoughtful design and testing was put into this one piece of art.

Michal Stawicki, habit coach, author of *The Art of Persistence* and *Making Business Connections That Count*

If you're looking for a book about the philosophy of habit-forming, this is possibly the most comprehensive one you will find.

Amazon reviewer

For anyone looking at gaining an in-depth knowledge of habit formation and development . . . there is probably no greater resource out there.

Jordan Ring, author of *The Action Diet* and *Now What? Getting Unstuck in a Sticky World*

INTRODUCTION

Tiny habits, big difference

Is it possible for an extremely lazy person to finish a marathon race? Can such a lazy guy obtain a PhD and publish several scientific publications? Could this sluggish man write a book and become an author?

The answer to those questions is not only a mere yes. In fact, for lazy people, such achievements are easier than for workaholics.

How is that possible?

Marcus Aurelius said that humans are creatures of habit. In such a light, idlers differ from hardworking people in their lack of particular work habits. Thus, a lazy life is a blank canvas, which waits for painting with beneficial routines. Therefore, laziness facilitates the formation of little habits that can snowball into major achievements.

Moreover, if you establish such small automatic activities carefully, you will no longer perceive them as work. With some knowledge suitable even for exceptionally lazy people (like the author of the book you're reading), you can make formation and cultivation of the beneficial habit as easy as doing nothing. Passing you this knowledge is the chief objective of this book.

But what if you're not lazy? Could you still benefit from reading this book?

The answer is absolutely. Formation of beneficial habits you love to perform is the easiest way to create the lifestyle of your dreams and to achieve anything you want and need. Unless you have a perfect life, you can use the information presented in this book to improve your life, whether you are lazy or not.

Yes, I have to admit that if you are not lazy, you need to work slightly more, as in order to create beneficial habits, you have to eliminate the slave-type actions you already routinely do. You simply must release resources from your old, bad habits to make some space on your life's canvas. No shortcuts exist. You cannot expand day beyond twenty-four hours. However, if you are not lazy, you should gladly accept a short-term, additional effort to improve your long-term efficiency. After all, you are not afraid of work, are you?

But what if you have previously failed to create beneficial habits?

Maybe you think this whole habit thing doesn't work for you. I have been there too, so I know it is a highway to a mediocre, unsubstantial existence. Luckily, such an obstacle cannot really stop anyone from succeeding. Unless you let it.

You, as we all do, change habits and routines frequently without even thinking about the process. Therefore, you are able to create beneficial habits to improve the quality of your life and overall happiness. It is just a matter of developing a proper strategy to take control of automatic routines. Yet only a few succeed in such a challenge. Many others fail miserably; in most cases completely unnecessarily.

From this book, you will learn not only the overlooked root of most failures but also how to fix it—even, or maybe especially, when all the old, proven, habit-related techniques have let you down.

You will learn about habit development from a holistic perspective. You will read about the approach, which in contrast to standard viewpoints, sees the establishment of an automatic activity as only a part of a longer process. Of course, habit formation is the crucial, final phase. But it is only the third step, which highly depends on the former ones that are equally important. Therefore, I will explain the importance of *picking* and *tweaking* a habit before putting any effort into its *formation*.

Apart from that, believe me or don't, failing to develop a habit is not the worst that could happen to you. Fortunately, this book is also useful to people who feel miserable despite (or often because of) the successful establishment of beneficial habits and who could identify with the question below.

What if you have created beneficial habits, but the overall quality of your life has decreased?

In this book, you will learn how successful formation of a beneficial habit can lead to a worse outcome than failure to establish a habit. You will recognize the root of the problem, and learn how to eliminate it from your life.

***

As you see, almost everyone can benefit from this book.

Don't be the person who misses the chance to improve life because of an illogical disbelief or a huge ego. Don't lose time figuring everything out on your own, and don't judge the book before reading it. Instead, be the kind of person who takes action when the opportunity comes. Read this book, do the exercises, and become a person admired for success. Take the control, build your power to establish beneficial habits almost effortlessly, and achieve all that you want and need in life.

But if you already have a perfect life, please stop reading and don't waste your time. Similarly, go away if you are not interested in improving your life with habit formation. Finally, throw away this book if you are not committed to putting in a small effort, starting with doing simple exercises presented later in this book.

Still reading? Let's go deeper into the subject of habit development.

CHAPTER 1
Basics

People often fail to form a beneficial habit

Let's face it. We all sometimes hate performing routines we consider beneficial. I know it sounds counterintuitive. But sadly, it is true.

Think about it. Many times in life you set resolutions, goals or other commitments. At least some of them are (or should be) all about beneficial habits you want to develop. You deeply believe these lifestyle changes could have a tremendous positive influence on your life. Yet after a few days, maybe weeks at most, your relationships with those tweaks are . . . let's say, not so ideal. Without euphemisms, you simply hate or leave them.

I have been there too. During my life, I have tried to form tons of habits based on the recommendations of friends and experts. If you could name it, I have endeavored to establish it. I had a go at tiny habits and the massive ones, including sports activities, diets, philosophies, time management tactics, productivity habits, success habits, networking and relationship habits, mindset creation, healthful habits, daily routines and more . . .

I was deeply obsessed with personal development.

Unfortunately, despite all efforts, most of my trials produced habits that did not stick. As a result, I sent countless envious looks to colleagues who benefited from the habits I struggled to create. Every single defeat was a demotivating experience no matter what the routine's nature was.

Does this sound familiar? If you have undergone such a hardship at least once, you know what I'm talking about. You can suffer because of a habit from sport, work or any other life category. Additionally, if you are a good man, you will instantly feel guilty because of your jealousness. And this exacerbates your self-esteem even more. It is a very tough situation and exactly the type I used to create frequently.

However, there is something even worse about the majority of those habits that I have been able to form. I have learned by practice that successful establishment of a beneficial habit often decreases quality of life. People do not think about it much, but I'm going to discuss this elephant in the room.

The paradox of undesirable success

Most habits I established decreased the quality of my life. Paradoxically, my life has benefited from only a quarter of the "beneficial" habits I have created. When I failed to forge a habit, it was disappointing, but 75% of the time I settled a habit successfully, it was a disaster.

I thought that it could not be normal, and I simply must be underdeveloped somehow. But everyone I have asked has had similar problems. Therefore, I have dug through countless books and websites . . . only to find that the issue is common.

Every single day, thousands of people make habits they hate to perform. In consequence, they create dissonance between what they think and what they feel about the habit. According to multiple studies, such a lack of alignment (even in a single area) negatively influences all other aspects of life. In such a light, it is not surprising that when people stick with habits they hate, their overall happiness decreases. And *vice versa*, when they establish habits they love, which are in alignment with their wants and needs, they flourish.

Unfortunately, people often stick with habits only because of inner discipline, beliefs in authorities' opinions, and finally, yet importantly, due to the promise of benefits everyone claims to get from the particular change. As a result, we often suffer as much by successfully creating, as by failing in forming beneficial habits. This is *the paradox of undesirable success*.

What is the origin of the paradox, and more importantly, what can we do to escape such an unwelcome fate? These questions were among my primary reasons for writing this book. You can find answers to them within later chapters.

However, before we proceed, you need a foundation to build on. First piece of this needed background is the scheme of a typical habit creation process from an open-minded point of view.

Scientific disclaimer

Let me state here a scientific disclaimer. The percentages presented in this book are based on my pilot study performed on a small sample of people. They are only estimates showing the pattern and should not be treated like verified, quantitative data for the whole population.

However, the quality of the hypothesis would not improve greatly by conducting large-scale research. The nature of the subject makes it hard to measure, as every person has individual definitions of positive and negative relationships with habits. Additionally, answers to critical questions in surveys are substantially affected by the cognitive dissonance, especially by the effort justification paradigm.

Despite all of that, central conclusions derived from my pilot study are correct and useful for better understanding the interplay of emotions and habit formation. I believe the accuracy of the collected data is sufficient for the purpose of this book.

Dr. Dean Ornish, in one of his books, complained that the government forced his team to prove that walking thirty minutes daily could be prescribed to elderly people and would not harm them. A lot of money was spent to scientifically confirm this obvious truth. Not to mention a significant delay in approval of a commonsense procedure that could help many people.

On the other hand, I am not giving you professional medical advice in this book. Besides, I want to share my observations with the world fast. Therefore, I have decided to skip the unnecessary large-scale research and present my commonsense ideas, even if the details are not yet scientifically verified. If you accept such an approach, let's move on to the scheme of a typical habit creation process from an emotional perspective.

The 3-step habit creation process

Habit development is a three-step process. The conceptual scheme of the whole procedure is presented in the figure.

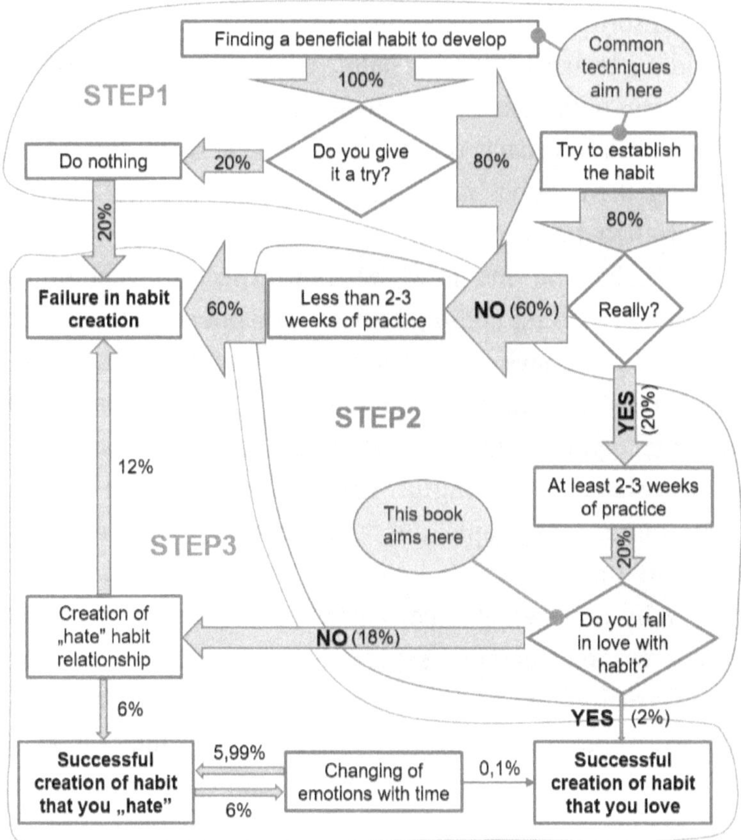

Fig. 1: The 3-step habit creation process

First step, first meeting

Let's dig into the presented habit creation model. Obviously, formation of a habit starts with the timely awareness of a habit's existence. At this step, you find a beneficial habit to develop: read about a routine in a book, learn about it from a friend, or get the knowledge elsewhere. Additionally, at this stage you make the first decision. You acknowledge that now is the right time to take the habit establishment challenge. Good for you!

Unfortunately, approximately 80% of people, after deciding to try to form a habit, do nothing substantial to follow up with their commitments. The widespread example of such an approach is setting New Year's resolutions, as writing them down is often the only true effort made to materialize the outcomes.

It's beyond me how we can expect to accomplish anything by doing nothing to make it happen. To be clear, it does not even have to be technically nothing. Often, it looks like almost something, but let's be honest. Could you always describe your efforts regarding habit formation as noteworthy and meaningful? Frequently, the answer is no, as three out of four people quit their habit challenge within the first month.

Why don't we pursue our habits of choice? There are many reasons, but one is especially strong. At the beginning, habit creation is easy. In retrospect, I was almost addicted to the early enthusiasm that always accompanies the first phase of the process. The promise of the healthier and wealthier life produced a nearly ecstatic sensation to fuel my effort.

It's nothing wrong with that the novice's excitation maintains your movement at the very beginning of the journey. However, accept that this enthusiasm persists and guides to final success only a tiny fraction of "challengers." Far more often, after the early spark, things turn to the dark side.

Suddenly, making any further progress becomes extremely difficult. When energy and willpower start fading away, you're doomed. It seems that despite the immense desire of a better life, you cannot force the path with sheer willpower. It is the illusion, as technically you can force the way. But the cost of such an approach appears too high in your mind and . . . in reality as well. This is a serious issue, but we will deal with it later during discussion on popular advice on habit development. Before that, let's go back to the model.

Second step, dating

The second step is putting the effort (either fake or real) into habit formation. The word "real" refers here to that feeling when you can honestly say you tried at least moderately and did significant work to change the *status quo*. Usually, a moderate effort could be defined as minimum two to three weeks of practice. After all, the thesaurus suggests "go steady," not "go wobbly," as a "dating" synonym.

At the going steady step, you create the first impression of the habit and settle in to a relationship with it. Like in human relationships, this courting stage can lead to various outcomes.

About 10% of people instantly fall in love with the chosen habit. This is the optimal case as in such a situation your success is almost guaranteed. However, with odds of only 10%, it is more like gambling than a viable strategy to maximize your chances to forge a habit.

The remaining 90% of people go down a different path. Usually we do not love the habit at first. Most of us do not like or enjoy it very much; some even hate it. This is an important concern, as it is impossible to consistently do stuff that induces negative emotions, without feeling bad (despite all the benefits).

Although various negative feelings can be involved in habit creation, their effects are similar. Therefore, for the sake of clarity and simplicity, I will refer to all negative emotions under the terms "hate spectrum" or "hate" in this book.

Third step, marriage

The third step of habit formation is the routine's establishment failure or success. Obviously, if you fall in love with the chosen habit, you will almost certainly succeed in forming the habit you want. On the other hand, if your relationship with the habit is within the hate spectrum, you will fail far more often.

Still, one-third of people build a habit they hate. Often, they believe their relationship with the routine needs just a little more time. However, merely a minuscule fraction of those people falls in love with the habit later on. Most stay with automatic actions they permanently dislike.

It is a pity, but this is how it works. For a similar reason, Western cultures reject arranged marriages. Let's learn from this example.

Such marriages, especially the really forced ones, work rather rarely. Often, parties establish a bad relationship at the beginning. However, sometimes they figure out their path to better emotions or even fall in love. Nevertheless, it requires tons of work with no warranty whatsoever.

A similar situation occurs with habits, but success is even less frequent. Part of the equation is that your family usually does not force you nearly as much to stick with a routine as with a spouse. Additionally, you probably care much more about your marriage than about any habit. But do not dig deeper into this metaphor. Instead, move back to the main plot.

Let's see what happened to two people (out of hypothetical three) who failed to form the disliked routine. At first glance, it is a huge setback, but please look deeper. These people almost always feel better than the early quitters, as they did not use low quality excuses. They remain mentally happy as they have a believable argument to explain their defeat. And they always could compare themselves to the "successful" people who are unhappy because of the habits they created, but hate. Do you see it? The only noticeable downside of failing in habit formation is wasting more time and energy than the early quitters. Right? WRONG!

This is what most people intuitively think. I cannot blame them, as I believed the same only a few years ago. But then, on one of those extremely lazy days, it changed. That day, I decided to stay open-minded and validate this belief.

Initially, I agreed with the majority. However, when I began to analyze it in more detail, something struck me. I noticed that comparing to others doesn't change anything except a subjective feeling about the situation that is an objective failure. I realized that effort justification does not change the fact that nearly 90% of people who put the real effort into habit creation fail either due to cancellation of habit formation, or establishment of the habit they hate.

You might think such people who put forth the effort must be the most logical target for books, courses, etc. In an ideal world, they would be, but on Earth, no one seems to care about them and their most prominent problem.

The vast majority of programs address wrong things. In some cases, inactive thinkers, who do not put in enough effort, are targeted instead of active doers. In others, the focus is on maximization of habit establishment no matter what. No one communicates the miserable effects such approaches create. This is a bit ridiculous, don't you think?

Don't get me wrong, such trainings are beneficial and can be useful, but have one fundamental flaw. They intensify the flow similarly throughout all the steps of habit development. Therefore, they increase the amount of successfully forged habits, but also the number of people who fail despite their effort because they establish habits that harm their lives.

It's just insane.

The overlooked problem in habit creation

The leading issue in the habit creation field today is that the chief problem for 90% of doers stays untouched. The 10% success rate remains stable. Success is bigger only in pure numbers. This means that the approach proposed by many authorities, experts and gurus is harmful in some way for 90% of people.

Would you take a magical drug that highly benefits the quality of your life only in 10% of cases, but has harmful effects in the remaining 90%? Maybe, if you are addicted to gambling, but I would rather do nothing than risk the status quo for such a low probability of winning and such a huge chance of loss.

I would lie if I told you no experts teach the second phase of the habit creation process. However, their instructions are not efficient and definitely are not designed to serve lazy people, who most of us are.

The gurus' tactics could be collected into two hubs. First is all about trying more habits to find what you love. The logic behind such a concept is simple. The more options one tests, the more likely one will find the optimal habit. It is, of course, rational and true. However, it is an inefficient (and sometimes even harmful) way to make things happen.

It is like telling a person to go to the forest and collect random fungi. After that, one is supposed to taste every type of gathered mushrooms to differentiate edible from dangerous species. Obviously, it is a foolish strategy. Not only is it extremely inefficient, but also hazardous. Indeed, many harmful mushrooms can be recognized by taste, as their flavor is disgusting. Such fungi are like habits that are easy to abandon after a short trial. However, some poisonous mushrooms taste good. Such fungi are like habits that initially look to be beneficial, but decrease the quality of one's life after successful formation.

I bet that none of you think that the "try all mushrooms" advice is worth paying for. So why the heck do we understand that regarding mushrooms but not about habit creation? Part of the answer is the slow and less drastic nature (compared to fungi) of the issues in the paradox of undesired success. However, to make the explanation complete, we have to add to the equation tons of stereotypes implanted in our minds through education, culture and all that nurturing. We simply prefer old, known hypothesis to the new, innovative ones. This is how it has worked for centuries for laypeople and scientists alike.

Thomas S. Kuhn comprehensively describes this issue in his book The Structure of Scientific Revolutions. While examples in his book touch only science and its progress, the core principles could be used to explain other types of revolutions as well (especially shifts in common thinking stereotypes).

I believe the book you are holding is revolutionary as it

presents a new paradigm for successful habit formation. Every new major concept challenges the old ones, but it also challenges you; thus prepare to fight with natural persistence to stay with what you already know. Remember that the old paradigm did not serve you in the past, and stay open to a new style of thinking presented in this book. And always test your assumptions in the real word, or better yet, test everything and have no assumptions at all.

In this book, I will not methodically explain the path that a new paradigm has to go to become widespread and approved knowledge (for those of you interested in the topic, I recommend reading Kuhn's book after this one). Instead, I will show you only practical steps to avoid mind traps holding you back on your track to forge beneficial habits.

But first, let me introduce you to the second hub of gurus' tactics, which is all about the efficiency of habit establishment. This collection of tricks concentrates on maximizing habit creation no matter how much you hate the change.

Following some productivity and psychological hacks, the graduates of such programs are able to increase the likelihood of success measured as habit settlement probability. It is cool, but the problem with this hub is similar to the previous one. It produces more misery than happiness as it facilitates sticking of hated habits and disrespects the size of the cost to pay.

It is like cutting your long, beautiful hair in order to maximize your weight-loss to look prettier. It's not only inefficient, but also a ridiculous strategy.

The promise

You may wonder why I am telling you all of this. I am doing it mainly because the amount of information belonging to the two hubs described above is overwhelming. In consequence, there is a great chance you are familiar with techniques derived from those ideas; maybe you have even utilized them in the past.

If so, you are not alone, as I have used many of those methods. Honestly, they are not that bad, especially when combined with the system you will learn from this book. So please, do not be ashamed or angry with yourself. You are not stupid, neither am I. We have just trusted authorities who teach the old-fashioned and absolutely logical information. Moreover, this knowledge was presented as if there were no valid alternatives or extensions.

However, the last part is not true anymore. In this book, I will show you the essential addition to the gurus' teachings that is actually more valuable than everything they have taught you and me previously. For many people, this extension alone will have more positive impact than all other techniques, tips and strategies combined.

In later chapters, I will dig deeper into the most overlooked part of the habit creation process in order to teach you a new, better and easier approach that maximizes both the probability of establishing a habit as well as the benefits that led you to the decision of habit formation in the first place.

When designing this method, I had in the back of my head those 90% of people who struggle because they utilize incomplete advice not tailored specifically for them.

This book is designed also for people who have failed,

even multiple times, but never agreed to be classified by authorities, experts and gurus into one of the two categories of their unwanted customers. When you fail, most teachers will tell you that either you do not want the change enough to sacrifice almost everything else (especially your happiness), or that you are just plain lazy.

They will tell you that laziness is a major flaw, so you have to change your attitude first, because no results are possible without methodical hard work. I am not one of them. Instead, like many wise people, I believe that laziness is the mother of all efficiency. Therefore, the ideal, most effective approach for creation of beneficial lifestyle changes simply has to be being lazy.

So I do not allow you to use your laziness as an excuse. In fact, if you're lazy, you have an almost unfair advantage over the hard workers. You don't have to rely only on your logical brain (occupied by common beliefs enchaining your mind) because you unconsciously feel what is efficient. Using your laziness, you can simplify and upgrade the knowledge you already have and cut the previous losses like Wall Street stars. Reading this book, you are already halfway into this positive process.

On the following pages, I will show you the habit formation system, which can increase the likelihood of success measured by the quality of your life and amount of happiness. You will learn an approach where your long-term happiness is more important than short-term results; the powerful strategy, which respects not only your resources (like time and energy), but also your identity and personal preferences.

This new method is simple to follow and will save you the otherwise lost time and effort. Additionally, it requires as little work as possible.

Don't get me wrong; some work is inescapable. *Perpetuum mobile* does not exist; and you cannot get results by doing absolutely nothing. However, I will show you the system in as lazy of a version as it can be without compromising the probability of your success.

I called the plan *Habit Launch* for the marketing and cover design, but it should be named *Stop Hating Sports or Work: A simple, lazy system to create beneficial routines that you love*. Unfortunately, the subconscious does not like such titles, as it prefers less complicated, catchier headlines without words like lazy or hate. Google the story of Timothy Ferris' *The 4-Hour Workweek* title creation if you are interested in extension of that topic.

The book's structure overview

In the first part of the book, you will learn the core principles and foundation of the system I have designed. This alone should allow you to make personal outline for better routines in life. However, in the final chapter, I will present you a step-by-step plan to implement the strategy with maximum effect and smoothness.

For the best outcome, I recommend you continue reading chapters 2-3. Then, while reading chapters 4 to 8, fill out a little workbook I have created to make the process as easy as possible. You can download the printable version of the workbook (as well as get access to other bonuses) at *http://moniuszko.net/habit-launch-extras/*

Without hesitation, let's begin the journey.

CHAPTER 2
Fundamental questions

This is not yet another habit list book

At the beginning of the core part of this book, I want you to notice that we will do things a little differently here. I will not give you a list of a hundred beneficial habits or routines you should try in order to fix various areas of your life. It would be pointless, as many authors have done this before. A quick search on the internet will give you plenty of such lists for happiness, productivity, health, fitness, well-being or anything else.

Instead, I want you to understand one crucial thing. You do not need another worthless list of the very best, little-known habits of successful people. What you need right now is one habit that is beneficial specifically to you at this exact point in your life. Every human is different, so it is your job to find this single habit. You might try countless habits from list books . . . or be smart and utilize advice from the book you're reading.

This book is all about creation and refinement of beneficial habits tailored for you—a unique human being. Stop pretending you're just like Steve Jobs, Stephen King, Salvador Dali, Albert Einstein, Leonardo da Vinci, Richard Branson, Ludwig Van Beethoven or anyone else. You're not.

Therefore, never blindly adopt someone else's habits without customization, no matter how great your hero is. What works for others does not necessarily work for you. You are inimitable, but so are your idols. Thus, what you adopt uncritically from others may work only for a short time. Sooner or later, it will lead to a catastrophe.

All successful people know this rule, so they often take from others' experiences, but never thoughtlessly. They skeptically *analyze* every new routine promising huge benefits. If the examination goes favorably, they *customize* the routine. Only when these two steps are accomplished do they put real effort into *habit creation*.

Besides, I want you to acknowledge that no one starts life as a successful person. What your idols do now might differ from what they did previously, at the beginning of their journey to greatness.

Often, staying on top and reaching the top require different means. Thus, do not form particular habits of amazing people, but apply their approaches to habit creation (starting from analysis and customization). In fact, everyone could get tremendous value from the personalization of habits and become extraordinarily successful. This book is written to teach you how to do it the simple way.

After reading this book, you will no longer skip two crucial steps at the beginning of habit formation. Nor will you waste time and energy on an unnecessary run of trials and errors. Instead, you will use all your emotional and rational abilities to act smart and develop optimal, custom-tailored routines.

You are special, so you need an individualized solution. Therefore, I will show you the strategy to sculpt your own best approach to form beneficial habits.

The importance of starting right

I know that extensive preparation before committing to an actual habit formation is not appealing. Nevertheless, such an effort is essential if you want to start out in the right direction. And I cannot state enough the importance of an accurate beginning. A single step in the right direction is worth several misdirected and a pack of random ones. Don't you believe me? Then look at the figure below.

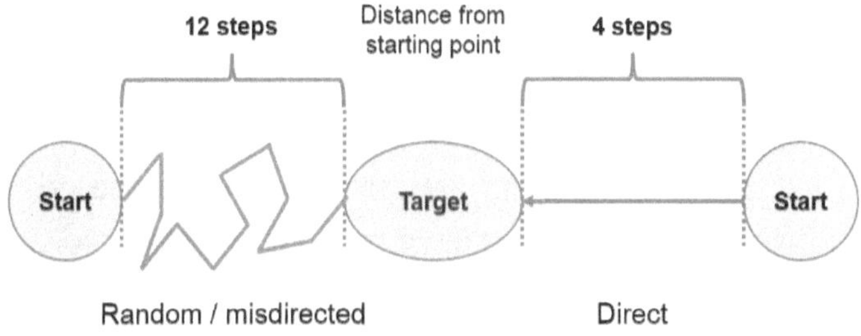

Fig. 2: The importance of going into right direction

Of course, this is a simplistic example. In the real world, direct route takes about five steps, misdirected ten to twenty, and random fifteen to five hundred (depending on your luck). Despite this inaccuracy, the principle is visible; looking for the straight path by studying a map can save you time and effort. Fortunately, you hold such a map for the habit creation in your hands.

It will help you to navigate from the critical point at the very beginning when the cost of every single mistake is the highest. Look at the figure below and notice that even a small change at the start of the journey can make achieving your target much more difficult.

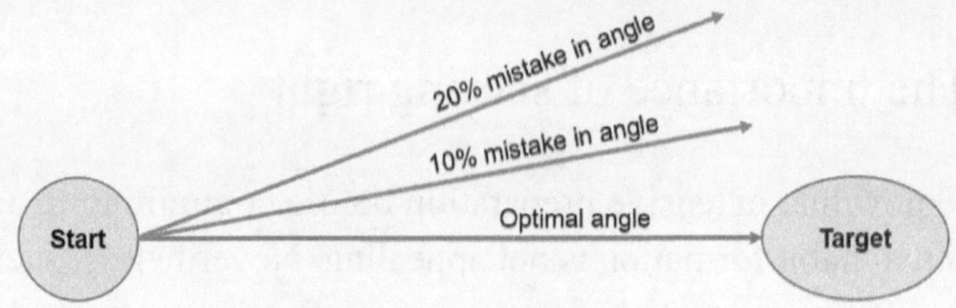

Fig. 3: The importance of starting at the right angle

Now, you should realize the immense value of an accurate beginning. Of course, you could correct your course later on, but it's easier to walk straight (or with only minimal adjustments) than to carefully maneuver your way out of a misdirected start.

It can be compared to a situation when you take a wrong turn at the entry to an unknown town. Theoretically, you can adjust the direction on the go. But in reality, you get lost and have two choices: look for more information, or return to the starting point. Either way, you lost time, energy and motivation. Thus, always start as close to optimal angle as possible under particular circumstances.

How can you ensure the right start of habit formation? By answering two fundamental questions before doing anything else.

Two fundamental questions to ask before habit formation

In order to make your individualized plan for creation of a beneficial habit, you are going to use one of the oldest philosophical techniques—self-asking. However, the famous questions like "Who am I?," "What is happiness?," or "How to live a life?" have to wait for another occasion.

This time, you will ask yourself two fundamental questions regarding habit establishment. Why are they truly underlying? Because the whole system presented in this book is built on them.

These questions are the keys freeing you from bad relationships with a habit at the very beginning of your journey. By reflecting on them, you gain the most out of the routine you decide to establish.

First question

First of these questions is: *Why do you hate a beneficial habit that you want to establish?*

Often we think there is something annoying or irritating in people, activities, or other things we hate. Unfortunately, we rarely recognize what this elusive something really is; especially in the case of habits, as the mission of correctly identifying the reasons for our bad relationships with them looks unnecessary.

Typically, we neglect the necessity of deeper perception into our state and want one solution to fix them all. But such a magical pill doesn't exist. We already understand that regarding health issues and accept that every medical treatment starts with a proper diagnosing. Most of us also know that in order to cure efficiently, we have to treat the cause instead of the effect.

Similarly, the primary cause for the occurrence of the hate spectrum must be identified for effective curing of habit creation diseases.

Easier said than done, as the primary cause greatly

varies from one person to another. It might be related to resources. You may lack time, money, energy, etc. However, such cases are extremely rare. Usually, such shallow explanations reflect the other cause hidden behind them. It can be some form of fear or self-doubt. It might be fighting with your core values or imprinted predispositions. Perhaps, it is as trivial as lack of excitement leading to the feeling of boredom. Alternatively, it could be your jealousness about someone who has achieved what you have not.

There are so many possibilities that only some sort of systematic approach can uncover the issue's origin, so often hidden under the blanket made of your beliefs, excuses, self-explanations and sheer lies. To make the accurate diagnosis of a primary cause, you need to remove this curtain.

How to look behind such a screen?

Ideally, every person should have a private mentor who is an expert in the field. But this is unrealistic. Fortunately, you can get similar results using the self-diagnostics described in the following chapters.

Second question

Second question is: *Why do you want to establish a particular habit?*

This one is even trickier, as our default answer has not changed since childhood. I want it because I want it—is what we think so often. Unfortunately, it is definitely not a decent response.

Pure want for its own sake is seldom enough to establish a habit. Usually, shallow desires do not strongly motivate us. Additionally, they are difficult to measure as you cannot truly tell how badly you want something unless it is an obsession.

But, you can perform an investigation for the more specific reason for your craving. Of course, such research must not be restricted to surface. To improve your habit creation success rate, you have to dig deeper and reveal all the components of your "want" whether it is a shameful motivation, childhood dream, pure ego, jealousness, or something else.

It is a difficult task, as we are usually more self-restricted regarding our "want" than our "hate." We can easily admit what we hate (at least to ourselves), but we often hide what actually motivates us. The explanation of such phenomenon is complex.

Concerning beneficial habit formation, usually there are many more things that drive us than things we hate. First, there are benefits we want. But behind the obvious things hide not so trivial ones; and after those, lay surprising forces, which we could not even predict at the beginning of the diagnosing.

It is like walking in a thick fog, when each step shows you details you were previously unable to see. It makes the journey exciting but also exhausting as no shortcut exists. But, for improving your relationships with a habit, you need to find as many components of your want to form a particular routine as you can; one by one.

It might look like a waste of time, but resources spent on self-diagnosing are well invested. The fact that you are reading these words confirms such a statement.

I would not have finished this book without a deep, honest look at a complex network of reasons to write it.

Not knowing my motivations, I would miss an opportunity to become an author. Instead of putting words on screen, editing numerous manuscripts, and publishing, I would do something else (like many times before), and stay miserable creating a hate-spectrum relationship with writing as a beneficial habit.

Synergy of fundamental questions

Answering the question of "why want" greatly improved my routines and overall life balance. But the real power comes when you combine both fundamental questions, as they are synergistic, which means that their mutual result is greater than the sum of their individual effects. However, so much knowledge, and the existence of countless possibilities to use it, might be overwhelming.

Therefore, in this book, I will show you a step-by-step formula to simplify making your personal long-term plan to create beneficial habits that you need, want and love to perform. If you do everything as described, your plan will assure victory on the first try in 90% of cases, shifting your previous high rate of failure into success.

Are you ready for that? I bet you are. So let's move to details beginning from a self-diagnosing using two fundamental questions you have just learned.

CHAPTER 3
First fundamental question

On the importance of strong feelings

Based on previous chapters, it looks as if the stronger you hate a beneficial habit, the worse your situation is. I have not written anything like that, but you put the most common meaning between the lines using logic and experience. All readers do this, including me. And it is solely a writer's job to clearly communicate the true sense of a message, especially when it is opposite to the typical way of thinking. Let me do this.

Our minds naturally link the strongest cause to the strongest effect. Usually quick making of such connotation is terrific, as it saves a lot of time and ink. But in the case of emotions, the strong hate is usually better than a mild negative relationship from the hate spectrum. That is how emotions work, and you already know it as I will prove below.

Unless you are a high-level Buddhist monk, your emotions tremendously influence your life. This is neither good nor bad; it is just a fact that we all have to face. This means that the rational mind is usually responsible for only a part of the success. The other part depends on the emotional side.

You are already aware that falling in love with a habit

of choice increases your success rate. It is intuitive and does not require explanation. What needs a commentary is the counterintuitive statement that mild emotions are almost always worse than intense ones.

How do we explain this?

Many rationalizations are possible, but in our case, the best one is based on emotional commitment. When we feel a deep emotional connection with a habit, we either hate it or love it. This is a desirable situation, as when our feelings are strong, we know that we care enough to succeed. Some of us even recognize the vector of feelings, but usually we don't.

In fact, strong hate blinds our rational mind in a similar manner to strong love. It sounds unreasonable until you think about it and notice that it happens all the time in the world of human relationships.

Look at the classical romances. How often do they explore a topic like this? The hero meets a perfect second half and for the next three hundred pages of the book (or two hours of a movie) wonders whether it is hate or love. I know I trivialize this serious dilemma, but please forgive my tactlessness, as my goal is only to show you how easily we can confuse the powerful emotions of hate and love.

I have another analogy to show you that this is not such an extraordinary phenomenon. Humans cannot differentiate extreme cold from extreme hot in blind tests. It is a *Homo sapiens* physiological characteristic and no one can overcome it because in a human's skin there is only one type of receptor responsible for perceiving extreme temperature. This is why you feel burning not only when you put your hand into fire, but also when your deep layer of skin freezes. However, without blindfolding, you can deduce the cause by seeing the overall context.

Often, a comparable situation occurs considering your strong relationships with habits. Either a love or hate attitude to a routine creates a similar, severe feeling of discomfort. Therefore, you can confuse these contrasting emotions in a blind test or with insufficient analysis. Bearing in mind the context, experience, and using self-diagnosing techniques, you could decrease the occurrence of errors. However, emotional relationships are not straightforward and stable, as feelings fluctuate and often dance in a pattern impossible to predict.

Based on all of that, before you can answer two fundamental questions, you need to ask yourself how strong your relationship with the habit is. Additionally, ponder whether you could make this relationship stronger. Such an analysis is crucial as a vast part of what you can do to improve the situation depends on the answer.

If you don't care enough about a chosen habit, you will always fail to establish it. Such a failure may take days, weeks or months, but it will happen. Trust me on that. Like in marriage; when emotions are cold, a catastrophe is just around the corner.

Fortunately, this book is designed to strengthen your relationship with a chosen habit. Therefore, in the worst-case scenario, you will be able to cut your loss immediately. When you cannot increase the temperature of your feelings, you can leave the habit, try a new routine, and still be content with the decision. But usually, that will not happen. Typically, you will love the chosen habit, succeed in the creation of a highly beneficial routine, and be enormously happy with it.

Reasons of hate outside the habit

A good starting point for digging deeper into the first fundamental question is identification of the reason for your hate. Believe me or not, in most cases, what you hate is not related directly to the habit. I know that this is yet another arguable thesis, but is there really a controversy here? Honestly, how often do you hate your habit not because of its features but rather due to your approach?

How often do you start creating your habit with everything set up perfectly? The answer is probably never, but the lack of precision is not the issue. The problem begins when you set up things in a completely unusable way. Your approach is usually closer to disaster than to perfection, and this is a serious matter as it could lead to the hate spectrum relationship with what might otherwise be a potentially lovable habit. Don't you believe me? Below I strengthen my statement showing some common mistakes. While reading these examples, please think about the negative emotional impact of the presented situations.

What would you think if I asked you to wake up in the middle of the night and do ten push-ups? You would think I'm crazy, wouldn't you? And you would be right. But when you start habit creation by messing with your energy rhythms or sacrificing your leisure time, you do not think it is stupid. Yet there is no difference.

You cannot expect a positive outcome if you bind habit formation to a time when you are in a bad mood. Or when you try to establish a routine during a time of day when you do not have energy and can think only about rest. Or when you trade your precious leisure activities for the illusion of a beneficial routine.

Stop deceiving yourself, and honestly anticipate probable outcomes. Otherwise, you might mistakenly hate your lovable habit by not respecting your weak and strong points, and other parameters, either mentioned above or saved for a later part of this book. In other words, you need to create a proper plan by excluding avoidable problems.

One such important issue stems from using too much willpower at the beginning. To keep your mind rolling, let me use it as a good example of a standard mistake (it may even be the most common one). Below you will find an analysis of the root of the problem and suggestions of how you can deal with such an issue. Treat this as a little demonstration of how you could walk around many reasons of hate when they are not direct characteristics of a habit.

***

You cannot win in the long run if you set yourself up for a sprint. Yet, you often train like Usain Bolt, but show up at the start of a marathon. In addition, you still believe that you will win the race. Anticipating success in such a situation is foolish, yet we all do this repeatedly. Typically, we start way too fast, use all our willpower early, and then fail miserably.

Common advice to overcome this issue is to develop more persistence. But it is hard to do so. We simply cannot change the amount of willpower available to us, at least not easily and substantially. So, are we doomed? Not exactly, as another way exists. You can quickly learn how to use existing willpower more efficiently.

Starting a new habit is all about consistency, right? So, in order to maximize the potential that the habit will stick, you should concentrate all your effort on regularity. This is an obvious line of reasoning. Thus, let me show you how to put this logic into action.

First, identify the tiny starting point of your habit. For example, when you want to establish a running routine, it would be dressing-up, going outside and running fifty meters. For the writing routine, it would be sitting in front of the page for five minutes. Such small commitments do not sound like huge steps in the habit formation process, but they are.

Running fifty meters or writing for five minutes does not require much willpower, as both activities look tiny. They are simply not a big deal for your mind. This allows you to avoid preventable will issues and to be consistent enough to establish a routine that you could always scale up later on.

This is already great news. But even more exciting is that after this easy start, you can freely choose (based on your feeling that day) whether to continue. After achieving your daily tiny target, you may stop writing, running, etc., without any bad feelings as you already accomplished the most important task. Or you can continue for a little while and do more, if that sounds easy and fun.

Just remember that no matter how long you write or run, you can get only one checkmark in your habit calendar. So please do not push yourself beyond easy and fun. Seriously, do not cross the line. It may give you more short-term outcomes, but for the cost of a highly increased rate of a long-term failure.

Reasons of hate inside the habit

After looking at the relationship influencers lying outside the habit, we can dig deeper into the reasons within the habit itself. First, you have to identify the characteristics of the habit of your choice that ruin your relationship with it. Next, you should start to deal with the detected issues.

Whenever you identify the reason of your hate inside the habit itself, you have four options. One of them is doing nothing with it, but the other three are legit: you can *eliminate*, *minimize* or *love* the problematic feature of the chosen habit. Let me briefly explain the process with the example of running.

Let's start from the last option as we have already covered some of that aspect. As I've mentioned before, when your feelings are strong, it usually means that you care about the habit creation enough to be potentially successful. In such a case, it is often possible to change hate into love. Going back to the running example; when you hate the exhaustion (slight pain in your chest, sore legs and so on) after running, likely you will love the same feeling after a while.

In this case, what you hate is often not the pain or the exhaustion itself but rather your current shape. In other words, the deeper reason is your present fitness level and as soon as you get results, you will fall in love with what you previously considered a reason to hate running. This is exactly why a deep vision into the truth about yourself is so crucial.

Another example is hating running because of the accompanying feeling of idleness. When you are jogging, you simply take the same step one by one, thousands of times without any difference. For some, it looks boring and disappointing. However, after a while many find running to be an effective type of meditation and fall in love with the same feature they hate at the beginning.

The second approach is to minimize the reason. For example, you could use your natural predisposition as an advantage. In the case of running, if you were born as a sprinter, do not start creating your running habit in the form of jogging. Instead, do a solid warm-up and sprint for a hundred meters a few times, adding some rest between repetitions.

Even if you are neither a sprinter (as you hate quick burst of physical efforts) nor a marathoner (as you find jogging boring), you can still run. Just do intervals with frequent changes of pace. Combine training with sightseeing. Walk, run, sprint or do whatever feels fun and get to know your neighborhood. Run with someone rather than solo.

The possibilities for minimizing your negative feelings are almost endless. However, all of them have one thing in common. You cannot remove the run from running. Therefore, if you hate running at its core, you have to eliminate the reason entirely. That means that you will not create the running habit. But don't be disappointed, as this is a good thing.

Remember that if you cannot love or at least minimize the habit's characteristic causing destructive feelings, your only valid choice is to eliminate such a habit from your life. Abandoning what makes you miserable is always a good decision.

No matter how promising the potential benefits are, accept that those promises will never come true if you hate what you do. Eventually, it will all collapse. And it is much better to demolish it in a controlled way at the early stage than to invest a large amount of resources and cry when you finally have to let it go.

Elimination of a habit is not the end of the world. You can always find alternatives that provide similar benefits and work better for you. In the case of running, it might be cycling, trekking, Nordic walking or anything else you love.

***

At this moment, you may feel a bit disappointed as I didn't tell you how exactly to go deeper into the "why hate" question to find what works for you. It is all for a purpose and according to plan.

Do not worry; you will know what to do when the time comes. Until then, you simply need the next level of the foundation. For now, let's dig into the introduction to the second fundamental question, which is "why want."

CHAPTER 4
Second question and pretesting a habit

Pretesting your habit of choice

Before fully committing to forming the habit, you should pretest it to see whether it is the correct choice. To do so, please download the pretest worksheet available as a part of a free workbook at *http://moniuszko.net/habit-launch-extras/*. Then, follow instructions from this chapter and fill out the form. Once you've finished the pretesting exercise, you will also have a rough draft of characteristics related to your desired routine. Such a list will be invaluable for getting the most from the subsequent chapters.

Obvious and hidden benefits

Answering questions regarding the reasons hidden behind your wants is usually more difficult than digging for an origin of your hate relationship with the chosen habit. However, the first step is easier as you should only identify the benefits of your habit of choice.

At this stage, you will find obvious reasons and shallow needs for pursuing the routine. They are easy to identify by quickly answering: *Why do you want to establish such a habit?* Take this crucial step now. Do not overthink and finish in under five minutes.

***

After listing obvious benefits, create another list. Making this one will take more time and effort as you will dig deeper into what drives you toward the habit. For example, when you want to establish a running habit, the obvious benefit is improved health and stamina. But plenty of other benefits might hide behind the desire. You might want to create outcomes such as:

- a topic for conversation with friends
- a slim body to impress others
- less pain in your back

Of course, these examples are just a start, as maybe you secretly aspire to be a marathon finisher or to compete with others (or with your own weaknesses) and have a great chance to win. Or perhaps you want to form a running habit to routinely pause and clear your mind. Whatever your personal hidden reason is, note it.

Please cover all benefits you can think of, as every desired outcome added to the list increases your chances of success. Thus, do not restrict your creativity, look for even the most crazy benefits, and do not judge anything at this point. No one is looking, so allow yourself to note unnecessary, additional stupidities and remember it is more important to cover as many things as you can than to do it exactly right.

Motivations

After identifying all benefits, your job is to disclose your often hidden, more general motivations for particular habit formation. Look at the benefits one by one and try to classify them into one (or more) of the categories and subcategories described below.

1. Achiever's motivations
   - Challenge: What motivates you are difficulties, obstacles and other challenges that allow you to perform at your best. You are driven by big goals and never quit because of temporary failures.
   - Excelling: What motivates you is not only the ambitious final goal but also all the tasks during the journey. You want to deliver your best-quality work, at every step of the process. You want to meet, or go above, expectations; your own and those set up by others.
   - Ownership: You want to control yourself and influence others. You want to make your own decisions and willingly accept the responsibility.
   - Pressure: You need some sort of push to perform at your best. You believe that some stresses motivate you.
   - Problem solving: You see problems as opportunities to do your best. You find satisfaction in finding solutions and creating a realistic plan to resolve conflicts and issues.

2. Builder's motivations
   - Developing Others: You like helping others to become better. You want to offer advice, constructive criticism, guidance, mentoring, etc., especially to your close circle of colleagues.
   - Friendship: You want to connect with people important to you on a highly rewarding level. You want to maintain a close relationship with a network of trusted friends. You want to feel they are here to help you, as well as they do not hesitate to seek your

help when needed.

- Purpose: You want to get behind a cause you believe in. You want to align your life with deeper meaning, vision and mission.
- Service: You want to sacrifice yourself, giving your service to others. You feel a moral obligation to help people around you before thinking about yourself.
- Social Responsibility: You want to influence others to understand social, political, economic (and similar) problems. A particular ethical or political school of thought often drives your choices.
- Teamwork: You want to work in a team and get credit as a team. You believe that a team effort is better than the work of a single person.

3. Caregiver's motivations

- Empathy: You want to understand other people fully. You listen carefully to their emotions and try to see the situation from their perspective.
- Family: You want to make your family a priority. You want to create as much love for your family as possible.
- Fun: You want to enjoy what you do, who you connect with, and everything else around you. You highly value optimism and humor and often make others smile.

4. Reward-driven person's motivations

- Money: You want money. However, often your desire is not for the sake of money itself. You might want material goods to increase freedom, safety, power, personal value, etc.
- Prestige: You want the respect of others. You actively seek titles, highly regarded job positions

and other visual characteristics of status.

- Recognition: You want to be acknowledged by others. When your good work is not appreciated, you feel demotivation and unfairness.

5. Thinker's motivations

- Autonomy: You want to be your own boss. You prefer working solo to being a part of a team. You desire the freedom and do not like rules created by others.
- Creativity: You want to experiment and discover your own, new way to do the work. You never follow the plan created by others mindlessly. Instead, you constantly seek improvements by adding your creative voice.
- Excitement: What motivates you is the risk and adrenaline. On the other hand, you feel miserable when you are forced to do the same boring thing over and over.
- Impact: You want to create positive impact in life. You want to do important work related to your life purpose. On the other hand, you are discouraged if your efforts do not lead to visible, positive outcomes.
- Learning: You always seek more knowledge. Gaining information might be a goal of its own or you could implement what you learn in your work/life.
- Variety: You want to change everything (responsibilities, routines, tasks, projects; to name a few) around you frequently. Even the smallest form of stagnation demotivates you in an inadequately huge manner.

***

I took the above classes from the book *What Motivates Me* in which authors Adrian Gostick and Chester Elton identified twenty-three chief human motivators by asking 850,000 people a specific set of questions. Therefore, in most cases, it is easy to organize your benefits under these categories. However, if you cannot find a match for some of your benefits, just put them under the "others" tag. We will deal with them in later chapters.

***

Knowledge of general, deep motivations hidden behind particular desire is extremely useful. However, as an additional exercise, you might also investigate for motivators you mostly identify with in your entire life. Optimally, read the book mentioned above and take the online assessment. Of course, you could also do it without the book, but I do not recommend such an approach as this is not an easy task. However, it is your life and your decision. Just remember one little restriction. You may pick your main motivations from only up to two primary categories above (ideally, 75% should be from a single category).

Why should you consider determining your main personal motivations? Because such knowledge is useful. For example, during the optimization step, you can incorporate those core motivations into your habit of choice. However, this step is supplementary, as it is complicated and requires Gostick and Elton's book to ensure the correct start. Therefore, I will not discuss it further during the optimization part of this book. Instead, I will concentrate on easier techniques that can provide as much value.

Costs

After you've clarified benefits and deeper motivations, you are ready to identify the costs of habit creation. The obvious costs are time, energy and related resources. Also, notice that when you do not create a habit that either saves or earns money, it usually consumes your cash.

Just remember that sometimes in the long run, you actually save even if your short-term spending pattern looks like wasting money. Healthful habits are good examples. They might cost you at the beginning, but you would save on medical procedures and pills later. Acknowledge that, but generally do not mix different benefits with different costs. Instead, identify the costs and do not rationalize them.

Additionally, don't forget about the often underestimated cost of better alternatives and lost opportunities. However, if your habit of choice does not directly interfere with the latter, or use resources necessary to do them, do not overestimate the price to pay. Just be honest and ask yourself whether your new habit really affects those lost opportunities. Will you chase them if you do not pursue a habit?

From my experience, it's rarely the case. On the other hand, you should actively look for better alternatives and always do what seems the best for you, right now and in the long run.

Cost of Inaction

Another often overlooked, long-term cost derives from the lack of habit establishment. It has a quite complicated nature, but I will present you the simplified version. This special cost occurs because choosing to take no action is not always a neutral decision.

Don't get me wrong; usually it is, but sometimes by not moving today, you will create inevitable costs in your future life. For example, if you constantly gain weight due to fat accumulation, you will have to pay a price if nothing changes.

On the other hand, you already know that the best way to improve many aspects of your life, including weight and fitness level, is to create healthy habits. Therefore, take into account the long-term cost of your actions as described before, but also estimate the long-term cost of your inaction.

Think about those TV shows in which people see their projected look after twenty years if they do not create beneficial habits (usually eating, exercising and socializing). Without doing a similar estimation, you might miss the actual significance of not taking action today. Because of your improper analysis, you might procrastinate and suffer by paying a cost you could have easily prevented. Don't let it happen. Remember that sometimes by staying in place, you indeed move backward.

One more concern about the cost of inaction needs to be resolved before you can go further. The cost of inaction is NOT one of the costs of habit establishment. Therefore, never add it to your list of costs. Instead, put it onto the motivations list to reflect its real significance.

Lazy validation

Once you have costs, benefits and motivations in place, you can validate your habit of choice. Most people try to compare against a solid alternative, but please wait a moment before doing that. While we will cover a similar approach later, this time I would like to introduce a preliminary step to ensure you do not invest energy unnecessarily.

First, you should analyze your habit of choice against doing nothing. This is important, because even if your habit wins over weaker alternatives, it could still be worse than doing nothing. In such a case, the chosen habit will be extremely difficult to establish. Therefore, always start with testing against doing nothing.

How to do such an evaluation? First, make a list of benefits and costs of doing nothing. It's easy. The benefits are usually either a lack of resource consumption, or what you could do with those free assets (like going out with friends using the saved time and money). On the other hand, the costs are lost benefits, bad feelings and so on.

Remember not to restrict yourself to short-term outcomes here. Imagine how you would benefit or lose out from doing nothing or performing the habit for a longer period (usually you should consider at least a year). Additionally, remember to include the previously mentioned cost of inaction as the important cost of doing nothing, if applicable to your situation.

***

Do not rush yourself. It's not a race. Do not focus only on the end goal, but also concentrate on enjoying the journey. Life takes place all the time, so it is not wise to get the most from it only sporadically. This point is very important to your happiness. Please consider it for the next ten minutes and note any ideas that come to you, especially those regarding the habit you want to create. Make sure that the desired routine has the potential to increase the value of your time, and in consequence, your life. You deserve the best, so aim high.

***

After creating lists for the chosen habit and for doing nothing, put the pretest worksheet aside for a moment. Don't worry; later you will use what you have created.

Reminder

Do NOT proceed until you have filled out the pretest worksheet. Seriously; do it now, or you will miss the opportunity to deeply benefit from reading subsequent chapters.

CHAPTER 5
Pyramid of needs

One of the most important features of the habit of your choice is its connection to your general needs. In order to identify those links, start by identifying and segregating your universal needs. Nowadays, such a classification is usually visualized in the shape of a pyramid with the most fundamental levels of human needs at the bottom and the higher needs on top.

Although the composition and arrangement of levels is a more individualized matter than some amateur psychologists say, the actual categories of needs are similar for all people. The most common pattern is related to the psychological concept known as Abraham Maslow's Hierarchy of Needs.

The Maslow's model is a good general scheme you can likely relate to. However, remember it is non-individualized, which means that the detailed picture of the pyramid varies (often substantially) from one person to another. With that in mind, look at the figure below and read the short description of the most widespread model of a pyramid classifying general human needs.

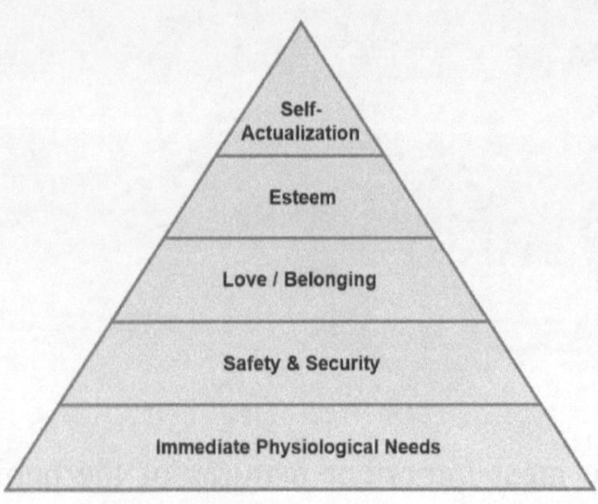

Fig. 4: Classic pyramid of needs

Maslow identified five levels of human needs. At the bottom three levels of his pyramid lie so-called *deficiency needs*, starting from the basic physiological needs. More advanced needs, also known as *growth needs*, sit at the top (fourth and fifth section). The basic description of each layer is presented below.

Immediate Physiological Needs are at the lowest level. At the base of the pyramid lie things like breathing, food, sleep, water, movement and shelter. If your routines do not already cover such fundamental desires, you should not pursue unrelated habits until you fix these issues.

Always start with what matters the most in the present, and then build on that solid foundation. If you do not provide yourself enough nutrients, sleep and basic movement, expect major difficulties in formation of more advanced habits.

The general rule is that if you have not covered the basic needs yet, it will be almost impossible to pursue something at a higher level of the pyramid. However, the threshold to pass is personal and can change during the life of a person.

For example, my wife cannot think about anything other than food when she's hungry. Therefore, for her, it is necessary to establish the habit of smart, regular eating before she can even think about higher routines. On the other hand, I can starve myself for up to forty-eight hours without negative influences on other areas of my life.

Safety lies on the second level of the pyramid. You need to feel safe and secure regarding your life to move on to the next layer. Again, the amount of assurance that you need is personal and greatly depends on your situation and beliefs.

You may be convinced you need a huge house, hefty income, great body condition and various material resources. Or you could be satisfied with much less. Personally, I recommend the minimalistic, stoic mindset that allows appreciating what you have in life and cures some common Western diseases. Additionally, every decrease in your basic needs lets you proceed a bit sooner to more advanced desires.

Love, understood as affection and belonging, lies on the middle level. Usually the need for love is categorized into classes such as sexual intimacy, family, friendship, belonging to various groups, etc.

Again, how much love you need to slip to the next layer is a personal matter. However, if you want to thrive in your life, you will need a lot of love. While in the case of material needs I recommended minimalism, concerning love I strongly suggest taking a maximalist approach.

Esteem lies on the fourth level. After a closer look, it is clear that half of the standard entries in this category derive directly from the love you experience. Here you find self-esteem, which is proportional to the strength of your love for yourself; and respect (for others and of others), which is also strongly related to love.

Obviously, you had better maximize the amount of love in your life. However, love alone is not enough to pass the threshold of the esteem category. The reason for that is the existence of non-love-driven entries like achievements, confidence, etc. at this section of the hierarchy of needs.

Self-Actualization occupies the top of the pyramid. At this fifth level, lies your motivation to reach personal potential. Self-Actualization is a complex topic that covers such qualities as morality, creativity, spontaneity, problem solving, the lack of prejudice, efficient perception of reality (acceptance of facts, self, others, nature), etc. The full explanation of all the nuances would take more pages than this book has. Fortunately, you don't need so many details for the purpose of habit formation. The knowledge useful for routine establishment can be condensed into short advice.

The takeaway lesson from the top of the pyramid of needs is simple. Usually we all highly value the autonomy, self-expression, profound interpersonal relationships with other beings, and fun (understand this as the ability to gain pleasure from what we do). Therefore, you should actively seek the solution to maximize these four characteristics in every routine you would love to establish. In fact, if you do not respect these needs, you will probably sabotage the process of your beneficial habit formation. On the other hand, when you follow this tip, you can expect peak experiences, honest appreciation and other positive outcomes.

***

To complement your knowledge about the hierarchy of

needs, I need to clarify one fact about thresholds within the pyramid. You already know they are individual and fluctuate. But do you understand how that influences your efforts? Please recognize that what allows you to barely slip through to the top today may not be enough to stay there next month. It is a pity, but you can fix that with a simple solution.

In order to keep yourself from possible negative outcomes, while staying on the top of the pyramid, you need to remember the lower levels and perform habits related to basic needs.

Imagine my wife forgetting her eating pattern for a single day. It actually happens from time to time, and the consequence is always poor (euphemistically speaking). She quickly becomes distracted and irritated for a reason not perceptible to most people. This leads to even more undesired results. Finally, all of her higher activities are negatively affected.

Could you relate to such a story? I definitely can. In fact, I feel similarly, when I substantially disturb my sleeping routine. When I am sleep deprived, I have to use a lot of willpower to mindfully separate the effects of lack of sleep from other circumstances. Rarely can the benefits gained from a sleepless night balance such a demanding work.

Thus, I try to always remember the importance of taking care of all my needs, either low or high; and strongly recommend adapting such an attitude. Additionally, search for possible habit improvements regarding the needs in your personal hierarchy until you comfortably settle on each level. Do not take this advice lightly or you will always believe it is easy to reach the top, but hard to stay there.

CHAPTER 6
The need/want matrix

The want versus need battle commonly takes place in the human mind. Moreover, the existence of such a conflict has an enormous impact on the habit formation. Digging deeper into the issue is useful, and you can do so using an idea invented specially for this book. The concept is called the Desire Quadrants, and illustrates four possible combinations of the nature of desire.

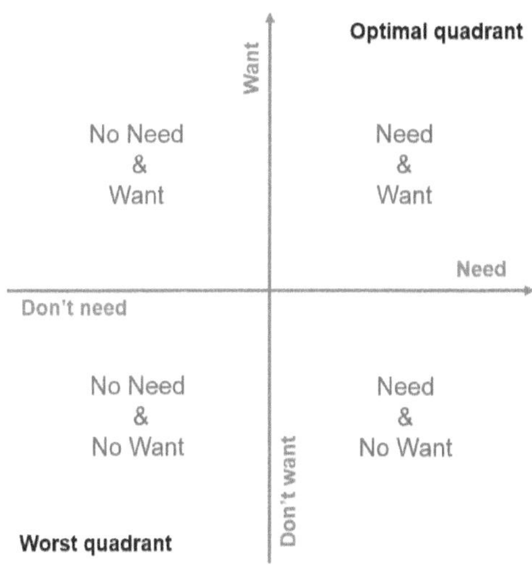

Fig. 5: The need/want matrix

As you see in the figure above, when it comes to creating the chosen habit you can:

- Solely want

- Exclusively need

- Not need and not want

- Want and need to form the habit

Optimal desire quadrant

The upper right quadrant is optimal for habit creation. An ideal situation occurs when two conditions are in place: you do not need any kind of additional, exterior motivation (apart from what is already inside you) to maintain enough willpower to establish the routine; and you objectively need benefits of the habit for your long-term well-being.

Need for a benefit is often problematic to classify due to subjectivity and dependence on the length of habit practice. For example, what you need might be a routine that enables you to change your mood from bad to good. Many habits could do that transiently, but hardly any could stand the test of time. The few long-term solutions truly belong to optimal quadrant. Moreover, only they could meet the expectations and fulfill your deep, objective needs without negative side effects. Let me clarify this in an example.

Look at the most common human habits regarding quickly shifting the frame of mind. For many women, the frequent way out is shopping. But the positive results of shopping rely on various uncontrollable factors, and thus are unpredictable. Moreover, shopping works only as a short-term solution. Later on, if you become psychologically addicted, it would bring more harm than benefit.

A similar situation occurs in the case of drug usage, which seems to be preferred by mankind. When a typical man is in a bad mood, he might try to improve the situation using a magical pill, powder or a shot. But neither alcohol, nor drugs, nor psychoactive medicines could serve anyone well in the long run. Again, they are effective short-term solutions, but can be harmful if used routinely.

I hope that after reading the above example you agree that the choice of a long-term solution is a more important issue than most people realize. Fortunately, it is the only serious difficulty related to the optimal quadrant of the need/want matrix. On the contrary, the three remaining quadrants are packed with potential problems.

The worst desire quadrant

The lower-left part of the matrix represents the opposite of the optimal situation. In this least desirable quadrant, you have so many problems with the habit that you should not try to improve anything. If there are no benefits you need to gain, and you do not want the change itself, save your precious life resources and simply abandon the habit without hesitation.

Please notice that routines classified in this section cannot objectively pass the validation versus doing nothing. Therefore, the only legit option you have is to give up on even thinking about them.

Existence of only one correct response makes this quadrant easy to cope with. On the other hand, dealing with the yet undiscussed half of the matrix requires more brainwork.

The two most common quadrants

The chief objective for habits in two remaining quadrants is to move them as close to the optimal quadrant as possible. Rarely is it mission impossible, which usually comes from unintended mistakes during specifying the position of the habit within the matrix. No one can be fully unbiased doing this type of assessment, and that is fine. Please acknowledge that such situations might occur, and do not worry when approaches discussed below will not work. In such a case, you can easily move the habit into the worst quadrant (where it belonged from the beginning) and give up the routine.

Moving into optimal quadrant

Moving habits into optimal quadrant could be accomplished by deliberate creation of want or need. Let's start with the latter, as it's easier, because when you truly want something, you naturally rationalize why you need it. It is a good tendency so long as your desire is driven by strong inner motivation.

If you want something desperately for a long time, it does not even matter if it's solely for its own sake. You can be uninterested in particular results, long-term benefits or any type of reward, and still create the difficult habit. Almost everything is possible when strong desire stems from your inner self. Believe me, it is one of the hardest mindset features to create on demand. Therefore, if it exists inside you already, do not dare to waste the opportunity.

Instead, enjoy this perfect situation and treat what you do as a thing you are called to do. It is easy as you already think about it more as a play than work, even when it requires a lot of effort.

Treat your habit like a hobby, which you want but do not have to do, and you will succeed far more often. This looks straightforward but the consequences are tremendous. Never throw away things from the upper left quadrant of want/don't need if your motivation is internal and strong. Such a mistake would be a crime against your natural predispositions, and in the long run, would kill the happy child part of you. You do not want to be a murderer, do you? So never let that happen. Instead, use the case to your advantage and create more needs around your inner wants.

Think about the wealthy person who goes to the desert just to walk through miles of sand and sweat like a pig. Similar situations happen all the time around the world. Notice all those millionaires who spend their time, effort and money on something that looks like a useless hobby. Is that crazy? In rare cases, it might be, but usually it is perfectly rational.

From the spectator position, it is hard to see what important needs are fulfilled by well-structured hobbies of successful individuals. In fact, ordinary people usually don't even care to think about it. Instead, they copy the approach of their idols without consideration of their own needs. What a misunderstanding of the whole concept that is.

Exactly like successful people, you need to regularly satisfy various needs. But you also have to remember that the nature of those desires is personal. Therefore, your habits, including leisure pursuits, must be carefully tailored. Below you will find some basic inspiration for using hobbies (and other strong, inner desires) to your advantage.

*****

Never underestimate the power of a true passion. Instead, establish habits you are obsessed about. Unfortunately, such routines might not work well straight out of the box. They simply may not give you what you need at this exact time in your life, at least not without some improvements. However, with just a few adjustments here and there, you can incorporate various needs into every habit you want for its own sake. Therefore, use all your mental powers to improve every possible aspect of the chosen habit.

Consider starting from the well-known fact that humans get more pleasure from active entertainment than from passive so long as they are not overtired and have enough high quality sleep, rest, and nutrients from meals. Similarly, a typical, healthy person values more activities related to the act of creation than those classified as mere consumption. That is why we can talk for hours about our creative hobbies, but only for few minutes about what we see on television or the Internet.

Therefore, you should minimize the consumption and passive approach to life, as they suck your energy and time as much as hard work. In consequence, you are tired because of your laziness. It sounds ridiculous, until you recognize that you can be lazy in either a smart or foolish way. Fortunately, starting to act smart is not complicated. Begin with making your habit more creative and active, as such a shift of paradigm would greatly improve all aspects of your existence. It doesn't matter why you have postponed such a move previously. Leave all of that behind you, and make a difference, starting now.

***

Another simple tactic to create more needs around your wants is to dream big. For example, writing is one of my strongest inner wants. In order to establish the habit of writing, I could choose various approaches to the very same hobby.

I could do some free writing, but it would not fulfill any further needs that I had. Perhaps a better option would be writing a morning journal, scientific articles or blog posts. In fact, I performed them all, gaining a better mood, more recognition as a scientific mind, and ideas about what people look for in a blog.

As you can see, small goals are good. But, only the big dreams can give you maximum results. So I sat down and wrote this book. It was the most difficult thing I have written in my life. In fact, my PhD dissertation was much less demanding. But despite all the struggles during the process, I deeply love it. Moreover, I know that such a book allows me to call myself an author of something substantial and that already feels wonderful.

However, as I am writing this, I hope the book will also give me some credibility, recognition and an audience to influence. Maybe I will even be able to push some people in a positive direction and help them create the better life they deserve. I am really excited about possible outcomes. Therefore, writing this book was the best goal for me, as it neatly combines what I need and what I want from writing.

***

Another simple tactic is expanding the natural tendency to rationalize strong inner desires. Just link additional, rational needs to the chosen habit and voila! You have a routine within the optimal desire quadrant to enjoy. Remember to hone needs from the low and high levels of personal hierarchy for the best outcome.

***

While creating needs around your inner wants is pretty straightforward, and can be done relatively easily, increasing your desire when you already need something is much more difficult.

The most common technique for getting yourself to want something more is the carrot and stick approach. However, such external motivation works well only in the case of basic needs at the bottom of the Maslow's Hierarchy. Additionally, the behavioral (reward and punishment) approach is effective for a short period, but it is usually not a viable long-term strategy.

Its performance could be compared to caffeine. A cup of coffee can give you strength and energy, but the boost will not last long. What is even worse is that caffeine is addictive and with time, your body gets used to the previous dose. In consequence, you consume more and more but the effect becomes weaker and weaker. A similar disadvantage is linked to the carrot and stick method.

Do not get me wrong. I don't suggest you avoid rewards and punishments or to stop using caffeine entirely. What I am saying is that for maximum payoff, you should use coffee and behavioral techniques only sporadically for a short-term boost in performance.

It is a good practice to always consider the undesired side effects, as they usually cumulate with time. Therefore, from the long-game perspective, the best option is to eat well to maintain a stable level of energy and use caffeine only sporadically. Similarly, the most effective motivation is the inner one with occasional rewards/punishments when needed.

Noteworthy, for some people rewards work better, and for others the possibility of penalty is what motivates them. Thus, check which type of external motivation suits you.

Trying rewards is simple; just make sure they are big enough to care. For punishment, you may use an approach that has been recently gaining popularity. Put some serious money (like 1% of your annual income) on the table and ask your friend for arbitrage. If you fail in your fellow's eyes, your money will be donated to the charity organization (by the way, the whole process can be automated using the website stickk.com). The trick here is to use an organization you deeply dislike. You should hate it so much that you would do absolutely anything to avoid giving them your hard-earned money.

The only thing comparable to inner motivation is a truly unexpected reward or approval. Even better if it comes from a person who you did not anticipate would do such a favor in return for what you did. However, designing such a situation is risky and unpredictable.

All you can do is give away a copy of this book to acquaintances, hoping that some of them will carefully read the previous paragraph. But you will never know the outcome as this is a chief point of the whole approach. Only a surprising bonus, reward or approval, gives the fulfillment and does not decrease, but actually increases, the inner motivation to follow the right path.

***

Besides the common approach of the carrot and stick, there are a few other techniques to create more inner motivation. One of the most effective methods is to make your habit more enjoyable.

I have mentioned that you should feel like playing, not working, during habit establishment. To achieve that, actively look for possibilities to improve the fun and pleasure factor of the habit itself and the whole process of habit formation as well.

You are the special one, so I simply do not know what you enjoy most. Therefore, I will not give you a list of possible improvements. Instead, trusting your intuition, I will stress only one powerful, and sometimes overlooked, area to explore.

For many people, it is helpful to create some gamification around the routine. Almost everyone likes at least one type of game. Therefore, if you can make a habit development strategy somehow related to a preferable kind of a game, the process would be much easier and pleasant. Such a scenario is solely positive, so I suggest constructing a game around your habit formation every time you can.

***

Another effective strategy is going for needs around the identified issue. For example, if you need benefits from writing, but you hate the core of the activity, find a way to get what you need without writing. Often, it is simple and easy. In the case of writing, try recording audio or video and literally speak your article or book. Later, you can even transcribe your recordings using voice-recognition software or freelance services.

As you see in the above example, the changed habit still enables you to fulfill the same needs but is a more positive experience. Usually, there are different ways to achieve the needs behind your habit formation goal, and you are responsible for choosing one. While you may opt for the hard path, I suggest trying to find an easier one. The simplest way to accomplish this is to create a habit that you internally want to establish, while preserving as many needs as possible.

***

Later in this book, we will cover more aspects of creating need and want around the habit you choose to forge. But before that, let me remind you about your uniqueness and the unavoidable consequences of this fact.

CHAPTER 7

It's the individualization, stupid

Power of co-creation and accountability

Another thing I want to cover before moving to the step-by-step formula is the power of creation. It has been shown there is a cognitive bias in which consumers place a disproportionately high value on products they created even partly. In other words, if you create or co-create something, you value it much higher. This phenomenon has been named the IKEA effect after the Swedish manufacturer and furniture retailer.

What does this have in common with habits? A lot, as in order to establish a routine, you usually copy systems made by others without adding anything of your own. Such an approach is a missed opportunity.

Instead, you can design your own version of a system for habit development to increase the perceived value. And, if such a value is higher, you want to use the created solution, as you deeply know it suits you perfectly.

Co-creation has another positive facet. It is the perfect precommitment. When you put some work into designing, you think as if you have already begun the journey. You feel as if you have already done the most difficult first step, and now your only job is to maintain the momentum. Such precommitment is great and often enough. However, sometimes you will need more accountability.

For that, inform friends about your mission, and ask them to check on your progress. This concept is based on your aversion to losing out publicly. It's a powerful technique recommended by many, but for most people it is not effective. Thus, always check how it works for you because statistically, if you tell your friends about your plans, you decrease the chance of achieving them.

By telling too much, you visualize all the outputs, and your mind feels as if you have already accomplished something substantial. In other cases, some of your friends might actively discourage you from pursuing your goals. Please take this into account when designing your personal system and think twice before informing anyone about your habit project.

The last two paragraphs are great examples of the importance of individualization. For some of you, I suggested informing the world about your plans and for others, I advised not to say anything to anyone. Everyone is a unique person, including you. You are special so you must ditch or individualize every piece of advice or approach that does not suit you out of the box.

The importance of individual algorithm

Putting effort into creating your personal plan allows you to deeply customize your line of attack. In today's world, you are bombarded with generic, best approaches to do things. But the solution individualized to fulfill your exact needs is always better than the ordinary version. Moreover, it's safe to state that customized is always better than even the first-rate generic formula.

If you don't believe me, look at Paula Radcliffe's running career. Even someone who knows nothing about running can see obvious departures from the optimal biomechanic form. Despite that, she is probably the greatest long-distance female runner in history. Moreover, when she tried to fix the visible problem of her shaking head or suboptimal (according to biomechanics) step length, her results became worse. How could that be? Is science wrong? Of course not, but most people do not understand scientific studies.

Results published in scientific journals are statistically correct and sometimes can be used as is. However, for the best outcome, you should use researchers' findings as a starting point for your own experiment to find what works best in your particular situation. Do you see a pattern? It is a co-creation principle in action. Start with what should statistically work, try it, and finally customize it to serve your particular case.

There is one more reason why following generic advice regarding habit formation usually produces mediocre effects. Successful development of the beneficial habit is a heuristic problem. This means no one can give you an algorithm describing what to do in order to establish your habit of choice. The universal approach doesn't exist. Only one strategy makes sense considering heuristic problems; you have to create your very own design of the approach, your individual algorithm.

Most people don't get it. They think that if something works for others, it must work for them as well. But such a philosophy is insane. Look in the mirror. Are you the same as the person you want to copy? I doubt it. Everyone is unique, and that fact has to be respected. Besides, you should not desire to become a pale copy of someone else when you could become extraordinary for who you are.

What you need is to make a personal algorithm so you can reach your fullest potential. Unfortunately, no one told you how to do that. But I'm here to help.

Simplifying the complicated process of creating a personal, unique blueprint to establish your chosen habit, I created an easy to follow 10-step formula. Such a step-by-step plan is the focal point of the next chapter, in which I will show you how to control and personalize as many variables as you can to make the optimal individualized system for habit formation.

CHAPTER 8
Perfect habit launch
in 10 steps

The sum of your habits is the most important factor determining who you are and what you do. Therefore, working on habits is the simplest way to improve your life. In this chapter, you will learn how to do that with the highest likelihood of success.

In order to see results, you will have to do some work while reading. It is not going to be difficult, as the tasks will be similar to the pretesting exercise from Chapter 4. But before we go any further, let me remind that you can simplify the process by downloading the printable workbook (which you should have already received after requesting the pretest worksheet).

In case you have not downloaded it yet, go to *http://moniuszko.net/habit-launch-extras/* and enter your name and e-mail address. After that, you will have instant access to all extra materials. Of course, if you want, you can continue reading without the supplement, but the workbook will help to ensure your success by making your work nearly effortless.

***

Initially, I planned to use gamification to make this chapter and the workbook more enjoyable. But although I love complicated plots, nonfiction usually does not benefit from confusing twists so desirable in fiction and games. Thus,

I finally sacrificed the idea of introducing you to the world of gamebooks when, after several revisions, I managed to make the whole process almost linear.

What is the takeaway from this story for you?

Remember not to be attached to ideas (yours or others') if they no longer support your goal. No matter how brilliant a concept (or habit) is; if it's not useful for your current purpose, just ditch it. Keeping that in mind will help you get the most benefits from reading this (or any other) book.

***

The original analogy to gamebooks was designed for you, my reader. But, I also had to create more fun for me. Hence, while writing the content of the actual chapter, I was simultaneously writing a fiction story. This story added nothing to the process that I wanted you to understand and learn; it was just for fun.

In the first draft, the fiction parts were presented at the beginning of each step and *italicized*. But those fragments did not look professional, so I removed them from the final manuscript. After that, I planned to share the unedited rough draft as a bonus. But it was so awfully written that I had to let it go, and deleted the file. After all, it had fulfilled its purpose.

You may wonder whether there is a lesson for you in the above digression. Actually, there is. The outcome of many exercises you will perform, will also be an unpolished draft. Do not worry, as it does not have to be perfect to be useful. You don't have to show notes to anyone, but if you want to create the optimal, personal approach to habit establishment, you have to write your draft.

Are you ready for some paperwork? Did you download and print the workbook? Do you have at least two dedicated hours to finish the job without interruptions? If you answered yes to all these questions, let's move to the work.

Step 1
Simple or complex?

You will start the journey to awesome habit launch by determining whether the beneficial habit you are going to create is simple or complex.

As you know, your relationship with a routine might be simultaneously positive and negative. You could simply love some aspects while hating others. Such dissonance is usually (but not always) proportional to the complexity of a habit.

An example of a very complex habit is cooking. One might like to fry but hate baking, love making breakfasts but dislike preparation of soups, and so on. On the other hand, some less complicated habits like running or writing still provoke opposing emotions.

Many writers say that writing can be compared to bleeding onto the paper. Sometimes it is indeed tiring and difficult. Yet, it is also so fun and rewarding that this almost masochistic part of the experience does not matter. The final balance is hugely positive.

Similarly, running can be exhausting. When you run a marathon, you do feel physical pain, but you handle discomfort with a smile. Like the saying "no pain, no gain," you concentrate on benefits and treat aches as a minor obstacle. You acknowledge the ache, but as it is an inevitable part of running, you deliberately choose to ignore it.

From my experience, the complex relationship with a habit is especially common regarding sports and long-term creative projects. It seems to be closely bound to activities requiring planning and persistence for peak performance and optimal outcomes. In addition, it's worse when a habit has many parts.

In order to fix the last issue, you need to split complex practices into smaller habits, routines and activities. Only after that, can you analyze them properly.

How do you know that a habit needs deconstruction in the first place? As a rule of thumb, it does if you cannot point out a single core activity as the essence of the routine.

A good example is rearing a child. It is not a simple routine, but rather a kind of a beneficial and rewarding work. The complexity of such a job is so overwhelming that you will probably love some aspects and hate others. In consequence, you cannot properly analyze activities like rearing children or even cooking without substantial decoding.

If the chosen habit contains more than one routine to learn and establish, accurate analysis of the relationship becomes impossible without deconstruction. Please go to Step 2 for basic instructions on how to do that. Just let me warn you that dealing with a complex habit is difficult. You need to remember to always keep the bigger picture in mind, which is often called a 10,000 foot view. However, you must pay attention to details too, as closer observation is also necessary to deconstruct and form a complicated habit properly.

Moreover, the above example is only a little teaser of the difficulties linked to complex habits, so do not pursue a complicated routine if it is unnecessary. Forming a simpler habit is the better choice in most situations, so go for a simple habit instead of a complex one whenever possible. By doing so, you can save a lot of time and effort.

For example, you will get the first benefit of choosing a simple habit by skipping Step 2 and going directly to Step 3.

Tasks:

- Check whether you can point to a single, core activity as the essence of your chosen habit.
- Decide whether your habit falls into a simple or complex category, and write it down in the workbook.
- Acknowledge that your relationship with a habit might not be exclusively positive or negative.
- Go to optional Step 2 (dealing with a complex habit) or straight to Step 3 (in the case of a simple habit.)

Step 2 (optional)
Dealing with a complex habit

So your habit of choice is a monstrous creature, and you are sure it is the only habit that will give you desired benefits. Alternatively, you simply cannot escape from it, as it is necessary at this point in your life. Either way, start by splitting this main habit into smaller, easier to "digest" chunks.

Please open your workbook and deconstruct your habit of choice. Let's say you want to establish a cooking routine. Then your chunks might look like: cutting techniques, boiling, roasting, frying, braising, herbs, spices, etc. List as many things regarding your chosen complex routine as you want, but remember that every chunk must be either essential, fun, or both.

***

If you have to do Step 2, it is usually a good idea to create a one-page personal plan for the chosen habit. Restriction to a single page forces you to be more precise and to remove all nonessentials, and in consequence provides more clarity into the formation of your complicated habit. Also, such a plan is easy to make.

Take a sheet of paper and write the essential chunks/skills you have to cover to reach your main goal. Additionally, note all the genuinely fun parts you want to incorporate into the journey. After that, admire the outcome of your effort.

If you need a visual stimulus, follow the link in your free workbook to download an example of a one-page outline. It is a simple compilation that I made for you after reading the "amateur part" of Tim Ferris' book *The 4-Hour Chef*. Please use it as inspiration for creating a personal plan for your complex routine. All you need is a blank sheet of paper and crayons, or some sort of a presentation software (I used PowerPoint to create the sample).

Usually, an elegant one-pager is more useful than an ordinary list in your notebook or workbook. For example, you might laminate it and put in a visible place to serve as a handy reminder.

***

The list you have just created is far better than the complex habit you had at the beginning. However, the issue is still overwhelming. You can simplify the picture of this complex behavioral change by making a main goal.

Pick a goal carefully as only a good one can force you to establish the habit. It does not have to be a difficult goal. So long as the road to the goal covers all the parts from the list of chunks, you are all good. For cooking, it could be three dinners with three various dishes. Just make sure the preparation of those nine plates covers at least 90% of the chunks you identified.

Once you have your main goal described, you need a flexible approach to get there. To start creating such a line of attack, just divide your big goal into smaller pieces. In the case of a three-dish dinner, the obvious choice is to create three partial goals—one for each dish. Using such a method, you will have nine mini-goals (one for every plate) to accomplish in order to achieve your primary objective.

Creating mini-goals might look easy, but there is a little catch. These small aims have to be built into a logical sequence. The first objective should cover at most a few (often one is enough) carefully selected pieces from your list of identified chunks. The second sub-target might use the already learnt skills from achieving the first goal and should contain another few chunks that have not been touched yet. The third objective might require skills developed while reaching both the previous goals and should incorporate a small portion of the still uncovered pieces.

The process of creating mini-goals is complete when you have fully covered all chunks. When you reach such a point, you could analyze the chunks (or mini-goals, whatever feels more appropriate in your exact situation) one by one as described in the later steps of this chapter.

Just remember that if any analyses you perform suggest removing the chunk, this should be thoroughly considered. You have to ask yourself if the chunk is really essential to achieve your main goal or if you could slightly change the goal so that the chunk is no longer necessary. Make sure not to ditch a complex routine due to a fixable issue with a single chunk or a mini-goal.

Additionally, while considering the chunk or mini-goal's scores, you should always be focusing on minimizing work and maximizing fun.

***

With your outline to achieve your main goal written, you're almost ready for Step 3. But before proceeding, take into consideration that your work with a complicated habit will take much more time than in the case of a simple habit, as you will analyze chunks/mini-goals separately. If you feel cheated at this stage, be aware that it is not me who has chosen such a complex habit.

I always recommend simpler habits unless you truly

need and want a complicated one before doing anything else. However, in such a case, you should want it enough not to be bothered about a little extra work to add a massive value to your life. If you are not ready for a serious effort, abandon the complex habit now and try something simpler instead.

With that final warning, let's go straight to Step 3.

Tasks:

- Split complex routine into smaller chunks (make sure that every chunk is essential, fun, or both).
- Optionally but recommended, create your one-page plan following the provided example.
- Describe a main goal (the simplest goal that covers at least 90% of the identified essential chunks).
- Divide your big goal into a logical sequence of mini-goals.

Step 3 – Looking for the origin of your relationship with a habit

Typically, there is an element of negativity as well as a piece of positivity in everything around us. Therefore, in order to rate your relationship with something, you should look separately for the reasons for good and bad feelings about it. Respecting this fact, you will analyze the origin of the negative relationship with the chosen habit firstly, and the cause of your positive emotions later on.

During the process, you will probably discover elements to add to the pretest worksheet. Do not resist the temptation, and expand the lists whenever you feel it's appropriate.

At the end of this step, you should have three exercises completed: I) the pretest, II) the negativity assessment, and III) the positivity assessment.

The negativity assessment

In the workbook, you can find a section entitled Negativity Assessment, which lists five main categories of reasons to have a negative relationship with a habit: inner conflicts, mindset incompatibilities, fears, lack of resources and habit characteristics. Your job is to fill those categories with all the negative feelings about the chosen habit.

***

Let's start with *inner conflicts*. Analyze whether a habit is:
- against your core values
- incompatible with your personal predispositions

Please list as many inner conflicts as you can.

***

The next group contains *mindset incompatibilities*. Look for beliefs that hold you back, excuses you overuse, low self-esteem issues, etc. Note them all here, but also look closely at what you listed as incompatibilities with core values and personal predispositions.

Please double-check that the positions on the inner conflict list are correctly assigned. We often mistakenly treat something as against our core values, when the thing is incompatible only with the principles we absorbed from others and has nothing to do with our inner standards.

Do not confuse fundamental personal reasons with something implanted in your mind by teachers, family, friends, etc. If you have any doubt regarding the nature of your negative feeling, list it here, not under the truly inner conflicts.

***

The next category is technically a part of the mindset group. But it is so common and important that I want to stress it separately. In this class, you're going to look for *fears* hindering your habit formation. Please list all those fears in the workbook. If you don't know where to start, below you will find some general examples true for most of us.

Are you afraid what others will say if you try?

Are you afraid of a failure and other possible consequences?

Do you worry about potential physical or psychological injuries that you might suffer?

I know it may sound ridiculous, but are you afraid of a win? Maybe, you are chasing the habit not for the outcome, but for the joy of hunting. This is an especially dangerous type of fear as it produces a lot of misery and procrastination. Therefore, make sure to spot this fear early to prevent serious consequences in the future. Such a fear might become a disaster if it stays untouched for a long time.

Are you afraid that you will sell out yourself in yours as well as others' eyes?

Do you overthink the endless possibilities regarding what could go wrong?

Do you ask yourself questions starting with "and what if . . ."?

Do you worry about unexpected obstacles you may face along the way?

These are all symptoms of fears that you should be conscious of. Such awareness will allow you to either decrease the fear's intensity or take the best from this feeling. But this is the topic of later steps in this chapter. For now, we will move to the next category of reasons to dislike the habit of choice.

***

The fourth category covers *resource scarcities*. Almost all of us lack the means to do something we want (or at least we believe that this is an issue). In this section, you are going to write down all the resources you feel you don't have, but need, to establish your chosen habit.

Usually the list begins with time, followed by money and energy. However, please do not restrict yourself to these. Maybe you feel as though you don't have enough relationships with the right people. Possibly, you lack other types of so-called human resources. Perhaps, you think you don't have enough knowledge or credibility to start. Potentially, you don't have enough accountability from your peers and family. Whatever your resource-related issue is, note it here.

***

The last group of reasons to hate the habit is the only one specifically bound to the habit you have chosen to establish and master. Please list here *characteristics you dislike about the actual routine.*

***

The above categories cover 95% of the causes of negative relationships with every habit. In the remaining 5% of cases, please put the problematic entry into the group that feels the least awkward.

After you finish the negativity assessment, you are ready for the positive part of the analysis.

The positivity assessment

In every negativity, hides at least some positivity. This is especially true concerning the formation of a habit of your choice. Every habit has positive characteristics, either direct or indirect. In this section, you will find them.

I am more pessimistic (or realistic) than most people. However, even I can find something optimistic in almost every situation in my life. This is just a matter of technique and knowledge of where to start the search. Regarding habits, the easiest way is to identify the benefits to gain.

Please write down as many obvious, *straightforward benefits* you could get by forming the habit as you can identify.

***

When you have your obvious benefits listed, write down all the *pleasure and fun* you could get from the routine and its formation. Put on the list everything related to the habit that feels like enjoyment. Maybe, you want to see your friends' faces, when you tell them what you have accomplished. Add such taste of success. Then, do the same with all the expected, enjoyable, playful moments. Nothing is too trivial to be fun or give you some pleasure. Therefore, write down whatever comes to your mind and feels pleasant.

***

Seconds ago, you listed the habit's *hidden benefits* related to fun and enjoyment. Now it is time to write down all other hidden benefits you secretly (or transparently) want to gain from your habit of choice. No one will see this but you, so do not be shy and move them all from your head onto the paper (preferably in the proper part of the workbook).

***

The last step of positivity assessment is classifying everything you have just written into twenty-three groups of common *motivations*. During the work, please add other motivators whenever appropriate. Also adjust the motivation list in your pretest worksheet. I hope you took the advice and used pencil and rubber; otherwise, print the page with the motivation list again.

Often, we confuse our drives and do not consider them as positive forces. A good example is the want of something for its own sake. Such motivation is extremely powerful, but could be mistakenly omitted. Similarly, you might feel guilty because you desire something based on a shallow reason. No one will see this, so honestly admit why you want to establish the chosen habit. Please think one more time whether there are any motivations left unnoted. If so, fix the issue now.

Some things are impossible to assign to the common motivations. In this case, put them under the "other" tag. In the previous chapter, I promised you insight into that tag. What you can do with benefits that fall into the other basket is more analysis.

Firstly, if you think that some entries from the unnamed group could be collected into a more specific category, feel free to create one.

Secondly, look at the benefits through the lens of your pyramid of needs. Take the benefit and ask, is it related to any needs in your pyramid? As you probably noticed, most of the twenty-three motivators are linked with higher levels on Maslow's hierarchy. But your habits often provide value for the needs from lower sections as well. Do not underestimate the importance of this fact.

You might need such low benefits to settle comfortably on the upper layer of the pyramid. It is a good condition when you do not have to worry about low needs at all. The simple strategy to achieve such a state is to create habits that simultaneously deliver benefits from all levels of your personal hierarchy.

To fully utilize the power of this principle, please think again about the possible benefits (from the entire pyramid of your needs) that you could easily incorporate into the habit. Write them in the workbook, and revisit them during the optimization step.

***

Next, answer these two important questions about your motivations.

Is the habit somehow related to any of your childhood dreams?

Do you desire the habit so deeply that the cost of its formation does not really matter to you?

Once you answer the above questions, your assessments are ready. However, you might need to bring what you have on the pretest into line with the assessments worksheet. Add these final touches now. In later steps, I will show you how to extract the usefulness from what you've created. Let's move straight to the topic beginning from validation versus doing nothing.

Tasks:

- Do the negativity assessment. Note inner conflicts, mindset incompatibilities, fears, resource scarcities and habit characteristics.

- Look for other causes of your negative relationship with the chosen habit and put them under the category that feels the least awkward.

- Do the positivity assessment. Note straightforward benefits, pleasure and fun, and hidden benefits. Classify your findings into twenty-three groups of common motivations.

- Look at the habit's benefits through the lens of your pyramid of needs to identify more motivations to expand the list. If some motivations classified under the other tag could be collected into a more specific category, create one.

- Answer two important questions about your motivations.

- Think about the possible benefits (from the entire pyramid of your needs) that you could easily incorporate into the habit. Note them to review during the optimization step.

- Bring into line what you have in the pretest worksheet and in the positivity /negativity assessments.

Step 4
Pretesting the habit of choice

As I mentioned in Chapter 4, validation versus doing nothing is the first test of value you could gain from the formation of an analyzed habit. In short, if something cannot beat plain nothing, it is not worth your effort. The examination is simple.

You need to compare your lists of benefits, motivations and costs of a habit and of doing nothing. How do you do that? There is no single answer as different options suit various people.

The most common technique is to *compare by feeling*. However, only a few have such a strong intuition that just scanning over lists gives them the right evaluation. Others (including me) prefer to analyze lists more closely and add more rationality to the generally emotional approach.

Here I will show you two methods more detailed than just going by your gut. You might copy, modify or ignore them, as these are only suggested tools to make the validation easier and more accurate. If you find the below descriptions somewhat confusing, please refer to the workbook for the link to a bonus article containing a visual example of a comparison performed utilizing the presented methods.

If you already use any structured decision process, you might notice that positive assessment clarifies the pros while negative assessment defines the cons of a habit. Therefore, you might compare a chosen habit with doing nothing using your current decision procedure. However, I believe the presented below approaches, prepared specially for the purpose of this book, are the simplest and most usable for dealing with habits.

***

The first method is the *Value Matching Approach* (VMA). In order to perform it, you need to connect the benefit entries from the habit and doing nothing lists. Each connection should contain records of the same perceived value (subjectively for you) on each side.

For example, if you feel that the value of the free time from doing nothing is the same as two benefits of a chosen habit, associate them together. Then, link remaining positions remembering that once an entry is associated, it cannot be used for other bindings later on. The analysis is finished when untied entries are left only on one side. That side is the winner, and the number of benefits left is the margin of victory.

If you want, you can perform more detailed version of VMA by comparing not only benefits but also costs. First, cross out the costs presented as benefits on the opposite side. For example, if the cost of the habit is lost time and the benefit of doing nothing is unused time, cross out the cost (but leave the benefit untouched).

Please notice that many costs of your habit should be reflected as benefits of doing nothing. Additionally, acknowledge that when the cost of the habit is lost time, the benefit of doing nothing is usually not only the unused time, but also what you realistically could do with it.

After removing the matching costs, proceed as described previously and connect benefits from both sides based on their perceived value. However, this time the process might not be finished when entries are left on one side. If any costs are left, connect them (still remembering to match the value) with benefits on the same side before announcing the winner and the size of the victory.

***

The second approach is the *Estimated Value Calculation* (EVC), which might sound slightly materialistic, especially if you are a deeply emotional person. However, if you are somewhat logically driven, it might fit you perfectly well.

To perform an EVC, write down how much every entry is worth for you in the preferred currency (US dollars, euros, exotic shells, or anything else). Don't forget that the value of each cost should be negative and put the minus before proper numbers. Also remember that for the most accurate result, the estimated value should reflect a fixed time; usually at least twelve months.

After projecting values of all records, simply calculate the sum for habit and the sum for doing nothing. The one with the bigger result is your winner.

***

Despite the methodology of validation, if the analyzed habit won indisputably, proceed to the next step. If doing nothing won, I strongly recommend abandoning the habit. However, the final decision is solely yours, especially if you've previously established several habits using advice from this book.

As a rule of thumb, never proceed with a loser during your first three trials utilizing the method from this book. Even after that point, be conscious about what you are doing by ignoring a warning, and notice that there is no warranty of success when you play against the odds.

The last possible result of validation is when your habit's victory is questionable. In such a case, strongly consider taking the mindset elimination step before proceeding to later steps in this chapter.

Mindset elimination step (optional)

As I mentioned in Chapter 4, sometimes the best choice is to eliminate your desire to establish a habit. In case of a questionable winner, you almost always could find a better routine to pursue.

You don't want to put the work into an unneeded whim or passing fad, as every real success is based on a long-term strategy. Therefore, look far into your ideal future life and ask yourself whether your habit of choice is genuinely helpful to arrive there. Maybe it is just an unnecessary, optional step in your journey. Carefully reflect on that.

If the last is true, usually you could eliminate your desire to establish the habit without reservations. In order to remove the leftovers of want, write down as many cons of the habit as you can possibly think of.

Look at the negativity assessment and appreciate the amount of work you still need to do on the routine. Acknowledge that this is not a bad place to leave the mediocre habit and switch to something more beneficial and exciting, with a bigger long-term return from the investment.

If you have any doubts, leave the habit for ten days. Meanwhile, proceed with another one. By doing this, you will check whether your desire can pass the test of time. You always can go back and finish the postponed process, but from my experience, it happens once in a blue moon.

Tasks:

- Choose the comparison method that feels the most appealing to you.
- Make final corrections to the list of benefits and costs if needed.
- Perform the validation versus doing nothing.
- Based on the result: abandon the habit, or proceed to Step 5, or go to the optional mindset elimination step.

Step 5
Initial cope with negativity

To correctly rate your relationship with the habit on the scale from none through dislike to hate, you must make your assessment as objective as possible. The most smooth way to do so is by eliminating what can be removed easily. Thus, in this step, you will improve your negativity assessment by getting rid of tiny mistakes that you have made because I advised you to put everything out of your head on the paper.

During this step you will also generate momentum, which is vital to get the optimal result from your habit launch. In previous steps, I advised you to write down as many things as you could, so you incorporated into the lists numerous questionable positions. Now, you can remove such entries with ease.

I know that it looks like a waste of time. However, the principle we use here is an old one. You might be already familiar with it, as it is analogous to a lesson from *The Karate Kid* movie. During training, the martial arts adept did things seemingly unrelated to the core subject (like painting a fence or waxing a car) just for practice of particular moves. You face a similar situation here.

The best way to learn a new skill is to do something not overly difficult, isn't it? Thus, you will begin to improve your relationship with the chosen habit by initial cope with five categories of negativity assessment. While making adjustments, remember that practice is the mother of all skills; the more you put into training, the easier later steps become.

Inner conflicts

Look at the first part of your negativity assessment. It has to be empty of deep inner conflicts. If so, you are good to proceed. Otherwise, you must remove all positions from the list. Eliminate, optimize, or walk around entries based on knowledge gathered performing both assessments. That should be enough to erase everything from this category. However, sometimes, a single issue might persevere.

If any conflicts against your personal predispositions are left, please add between one and three points to your negativity score (you can find a place to write down the score in the workbook). Half points are allowed, and two points is usually the right amount for a single entry.

However, there is a key exception to this rating rule. If what slipped through is not only incompatible with your predispositions, but a deep inner conflict regarding your core values, you "win" the additional *golden negativity point*. In such a case, please go straight to Step 7 of this chapter and come back when you finish dealing with it.

Resource scarcities

This is my favorite brake as it has been holding me back for so long. That is why I know you can remove most of what you listed here by doing almost nothing. How is it possible and what exactly should you do? Simply remember that your main goal is to create a habit and postpone other goals related to the routine, as you will achieve them only if you firstly succeed in particular habit formation.

In order to establish a habit, you do not have to invest

much money or energy. Usually you need no more than ten minutes per day. However, there is a little catch. These several minutes are sufficient only if you spend them on performing the core part of habitual activity you want to form.

Otherwise, you might encounter avoidable obstacles created solely by yourself. For example, I wasted a lot of my time by searching for and buying various Irish whistles (kind of a musical instrument) instead of creating a habit of playing. I made a classic mistake by concentrating on the non-core part of the routine, and then I reaped what I sowed.

It might sound ridiculous, but I created a habit of collecting those little shiny things instead of the habit of playing them. But was that really unexpected considering that I made a steady effort into creation of exactly such a routine? Honestly, it was surprising for me at that time of my life. Moreover, I am not alone in this, as according to popular Internet whistle forums, the Whistle Obsessive Acquisition Disorder (WhOA) is quite frequent and difficult to cure.

Comparable issues occur regarding formation of other habits. Therefore, I wrote about my story so you can learn from my mistakes and avoid similar problems in your quest to successful launch of your beneficial habit.

In order to use the advice and save precious resources, make your initial commitment to habit formation clear, closely related to the essence of the desired activity, and as small as possible. Want to floss your teeth regularly? Start with the commitment to floss a single tooth. Want to start exercising? Do ten half-squats and ten wall push-ups every single day. Want to be a writer? Set your goal at one short paragraph or even a single sentence daily.

You may think it is not enough; but nothing is too small, if you concentrate on regularity. In fact, I started writing this book using just five minutes as the initial goal. Only after I mastered that little commitment did I gradually move on to five hundred crappy words or sixty minutes (whichever came first), and I'm still on this level to secure frequent victories.

Going back to rating the relationship, add up to one point for any resource scarcity you do not remove by making your goal simpler and smaller (but no more than three points in total).

Mindset incompatibilities

The vast portion of the negativity assessment is about your suboptimal mindset, which holds you back. Fortunately, the issue is often easy to reduce. In most cases, all you have to do with your mindset incompatibilities list is to mindfully acknowledge the existence of the issue and recognize its true nature. You already know that those are only beliefs—not the laws of physics, but like many people, you might tend to forget about this considering your actions. Therefore, regularly remind yourself to never treat things you have noted as mindset incompatibilities as absolute truths.

Notice that your mindset is constantly changing, one step at a time. Every time you choose to stretch your comfort zone, you simultaneously learn new things. Those new insights slightly shape your beliefs. This is a slow process, but awareness of its existence is enough for what you are going to do in this chapter.

However, if you want to develop a mindset that will better serve you in personal and professional life faster, many books and courses could speed up the process. My personal favorite is *Maximum Achievement* by Brian Tracy. This was his first book and probably the best one (as he has admitted). There are more detailed and up-to-date books, but *Maximum Achievement* applies to the widest audience as it covers mindset shifts helpful in achieving success in multiple areas of life.

Brian Tracy's book will provide you with enough knowledge to get 80% of possible results concerning mindset. Just remember to use the information as reading any book (even the one you are holding in your hands) without taking action can give you only about 8% of the desired outcome. Speaking about adapting the knowledge from books, you should of course personalize techniques proposed by Brian. For example, many suggestions of Mr. Tracy suit my personality, but others don't; thus, I simply customized only the instructions compatible with my needs and wants. Always use a similar approach if you want to improve your life as fast and as easily as possible.

Moving back to rating, you can add up to three points here (half points allowed) based purely on how you feel.

Fears

Fears are good. It might sound counterintuitive, but it is true. When you do not feel fear, you don't reach out of your comfort zone and probably don't do anything meaningful. Such a stabilization is the surest way to a boring, mediocre life. Unless you are an enlightened, Buddha-type of person, you need to be afraid from time to time in order to maintain your feeling of progress and fulfillment.

Even experienced musicians or actors have stage fright every time they are about to perform. You might argue that it disappears with the first phrase of a play or a tune. However, this doesn't change that it always exists, even if just for a tiny moment.

***

Fear is a natural response of a healthy body to adrenaline secretion. I hope you can accept some excitement in your life. If your answer is yes, you simultaneously, unconsciously agree to take some form of a fright as a positive force. How awesome is that?

But you have to understand we all have fears that are almost useless to modern humans. The classic example of such an artifact is the *fight or flight response*, which is an automatic, instinctive action activated by various triggers. It has tremendous value in dramatic situations frequent in past eras when the choice was between life and death, but not nowadays when the possibility of fatal failure is much slimmer. Let's be honest; you will not die if you fail to create your habit of choice. Therefore, every time you feel an adrenaline rush, evaluate whether the trigger behind it is truly mortality-based.

On the other hand, you might fear something much less serious than death. You might even worry about something less important than starving, loss of shelter, etc. Your fears are very personal, and you have them listed right before your eyes.

Let me state something clearly. I am not judging your fears; you have to do that yourself. Similarly, you are the only one who can overcome your dramas. However, you can make it easier using various methods; from commonsense knowledge to complicated psychological approaches. There is always a way to decrease the negative effects of your frights, the silliest worries and the strongest phobias. You can master almost everything in life, including dealing with any specific fear. Sometimes, you will need intense therapy; more often, the general advice presented below will be sufficient.

***

Let's start with something simple. Please group your fears into two major categories. The first one should contain worries related to your basic needs. Obviously, everyone needs food, shelter and clothes. Usually we also need some approval from the herd, so if you are afraid of losing your family or friends because of a chosen habit formation, also put it here.

Under the second category, collect all the fears that, even materialized, will not drastically affect your life; unless you let them. I like calling them "silly worries" as they do not touch the basis of your well-being from the unbiased spectator's position.

Splitting your fears into two classes might feel unnatural. However, it is the easiest tactic to instantly decrease the impact of most of your worries on your life.

In fact, recognizing the objective importance of things is probably the most useful skill to learn in order to increase your boldness. People usually don't realize the trifling nature of many of their fears. A good exercise to recognize the unimportance of various worries is to visualize the worst-case scenario. Imagine what could happen if you fail and how it would influence your life. Usually, the failure will not result in huge changes. When you find that your basic needs stay untouched, classify the analyzed belief as a silly fear.

***

If you are similar to other humans, most of your fears are rather silly. However, occasionally your habit indeed negatively interferes with basic needs. If so, you have four valid choices that you could often combine into one solution.

- You could abandon the habit.
- You could change it during the optimization process described in Step 10.
- You could accumulate additional resources before proceeding with the routine.
- You could change your mindset to make the fear less relevant.

The first three options are self-explanatory. Therefore, I would briefly describe only the fourth route here.

***

To make the subject of your fear (either an important or a silly one) less significant, estimate the probability that it will materialize. Stop overestimating the danger, as you probably risk much more during your car ride every day. Yet, you choose to ignore those fears when driving. So why are you afraid of fears regarding your habits? You can choose to pay less attention to fear and deliberately concentrate on the positive aspects of habit . . . so just do it!

I bet that at least 95% of fears you have written will not materialize. This means that most of the time, you are afraid of the uncommon and unknown. You cannot predict everything with 100% accuracy, so your mind tricks you into procrastinating and thinking about things that will never happen. Instead of the habit itself, you're obsessed with events, which probably will not occur. It is insane and you know it. Fortunately, you need only a little modification to change such a situation.

First, acknowledge that every fear is present only in your mind. It is just your response to stimulus. This means that by working on your mindset, you can decide to not feel fear. However, it is a thought-job as we are already culturally preprogrammed to feel fear. We are not mythical Vikings.

Fortunately, there is a little trick to instantly make many fears less devastating. This technique combines the basic biochemical reaction in a human body and the power of the mind. Moreover, often, it is much easier to perform than fighting with a fright directly. I suppose Vikings could use a similar technique too. Are you intrigued about this secret?

It is rather straightforward. Just think about the fun activities that result in an adrenaline rush. They are full of controlled fear, yet you choose to perform them for the effects of various chemicals secreted and delivered to your brain. Similarly, you can cope with fears and enjoy them as a part of the fun and pleasure related to performing a routine. The skill is not easy to master but is pretty simple to start to practice. You just need a solid kick in the ass. And I will gladly provide it below.

* * *

Stop crying about your imagined fears. Move on bravely. Use the excitement you already have to embrace the new. Crash your fears with faith, hope, and at least a slightly positive attitude. You have to be bold, so leave your comfort zone. Otherwise, you will kill the joy of life inside you and become the walking dead. Of course, this might be your goal if you are looking for a mystical nirvana and want to become a high-level zombie. However, as you are reading this book, let me assume that it's not the case. You have to understand the weakness of your unimportant fears and smash them on the floor. Laugh at your fears. They are here just to amuse you. Like on a rollercoaster or in a haunted house.

You can't do that? No kidding. Why are you reading a self-help book instead of going to a medical doctor? If you cannot win with your fears, I'm afraid there is no hope for you other than a licensed psychiatrist and many pills of various colors and shapes. Paralyzing fear is one of the symptoms of a psychological disease. Therefore, if fear influences your life so substantially, your priority should be to strengthen your mental health.

Of course, I believe that you will pull yourself together and win the fight with those fears you have put on the list to explain your procrastination or for any other unimportant reason. If not, swallow your pride and just go to a doctor for a private consultation.

***

Let's move on to rating. You can add from one to three points here based on what you're feeling about listed fears after digesting what you have just read. Usually anything between half and a single point for every fear is enough, but the decision is, as always, yours.

Habit characteristics

What you listed as directly associated with habit might not necessarily be the problem. There are two categories of negative habit characteristics. One is extremely uncomfortable to deal with, and the other is manageable to walk around. Let's start with the latter class. If what you listed is not related to the core of the habit, please add one point for every three items you listed here (no more than three points in total).

However, if what you have noted is an irremovable feature of the habit (for example, you hate all type of running, but want to form a running habit), award yourself *the golden negativity point* and move directly to Step 7. After that, come back here and proceed with a slightly different habit.

Tasks:

- Rate (and write down the scores in the workbook) your inner conflicts, lack of resources, mindset incompatibilities, fears, and habit characteristics.
- If you win the golden point, move to Step 7.
- Eliminate silly, tiny entries from the negativity assessment that you mistakenly put onto the list. After eliminating the entries that are easy to cope with, adjust your negativity scores if needed.
- Note all other improvements that come to your mind during the exercise (and revisit this section of the workbook during the optimization process.)

Step 6
Rating the positivity

Humans are better suited to fixing broken things than improving something in working condition. That is why most sales letters concentrate on pain to remove instead of benefits to gain. Focusing on issues is the natural, default program of your brain, but you can purposely use other software on your mind.

To form a perfect, automated routine, you must not only decrease the negativity, but also improve positive aspects of a chosen habit. To do so, try to be more conscious and aware during three next steps of habit launch. First you need to *rate* everything you listed during the positivity assessment. After that, *analyze* your positive relationship with a habit and identify the vital points to improve. Finally, lift your habit formation to a new level during systematic *optimization*.

If the above scheme sounds like a solid plan to you, move on to rating instructions for each category (half points are allowed).

Straightforward benefits

Please add up to three points for the benefits you listed. Give the maximum score if the benefits are so huge that you desperately need to acquire them as soon as possible. Only a habit that would increase the quality of your life the most can earn you three points. Otherwise, you could assign up to two points here.

Fun and pleasure

Add up to three points here. Put the highest score when you wake up with energy because you cannot wait anymore for the fun and pleasure of practicing the chosen habit. While allocating three points for routines pumping you up is clear, you might consider such a high score also for simple habits that could create huge improvement in the quality of your life.

A good example is a healthful breakfast. You might not consciously recognize the pleasure it provides, as it's not directly fun. Nevertheless, a smart breakfast (with high protein content, some vegetables, some fat and enough calories) gives you more energy, allows you to hone your weight, and boost your well-being. It also ensures those results almost from the beginning of the practice. In consequence, it is a great habit, which usually deserves a maximum score for fun and pleasure.

Think whether your habit fits into the position similar to those described above. If not, allocate up to two points in the appropriate place in the workbook.

Hidden benefits

Assign up to three points here. This category is the most versatile one, so there is no good generic example to illustrate how to rate what you listed. I can only advise you to make it fast and not to overthink. Quickly allocate points by feel and just move on.

Motivators

This category is the tricky one, as twenty-three motivators you used as a guide are not equally strong for various people. Some of these universal motivations might actually demotivate you. Additionally, the strength of specific motivations fluctuates with experience and status changes. All that makes rating your drives difficult.

However, there are some general rules to consider. For example, if you identify more than several motivations, and they are mostly among one or two major hubs, you could easily add three points here. However, please validate the strength of your motivation with honesty and subtract at least one point if you feel uncomfortable with the maximum score.

On the other hand, if you find only a few motivations, or they are represented equally over the hubs, you probably should assign up to two points. However, if you feel that your motivation is so strong that you could easily establish your habit of choice based on that alone, give the maximum score no matter what. Using a strong drive that already exists is much simpler than increasing a weak motivation. Therefore, always respect the most powerful of your motivations and use saved energy to improve other features of a chosen habit.

Also, do not forget about motivations from the "other" tag. You could add up to one point to your motivation score if you noted strong "other" drives, especially those related to basic needs from the base of your pyramid of needs. Just remember not to exceed three points in total.

***

After rating your positivity and negativity scores, you need to calculate the results. Instruction how to do that is presented in Step 8. Notice that you can skip Step 7, as it is a "reward" for *the golden negativity point*.

Tasks:

- Rate (and write down the scores in the workbook) the straightforward benefits, fun and pleasure, hidden benefits, and motivators of your chosen habit.

Step 7 (optional)
Love it or leave it

You are reading this section because the establishment of your beneficial habit of choice will have a radical negative influence on your life. You have two legit options: eliminate the reason that brings you to this step, or abandon the habit and start the process from the beginning with a brand-new target. I know it is a tough dilemma. Therefore, give yourself a day to ponder on it.

Remember, there is always a way out of this kind of situation. It is just not so obvious and usually requires an out-of-the-box approach. As a good start, get more information by finishing rating your relationship with the chosen habit. Such an analysis will make clear what you might lose and what you might gain if you successfully form a routine. When you have this clarified, honestly evaluate how important the desired change is for you. Next, use all the gathered knowledge to create an improved (or a brand-new) habit that gives you as many benefits of the original routine as possible, but from a different angle or activity.

Instead of directly fighting, try to walk around the problem, which secured you the golden negativity point and led you here. Be flexible and crush it like Bruce Lee. I believe in you.

Tasks:

- Eliminate the reason that brought you to Step 7, or abandon the chosen habit and start the process from the beginning with a brand-new routine.

Step 8
Calculating the results

Negativity score

Let's start with the negativity assessment. First, calculate the sum of points you have given for inner conflicts, mindset incompatibilities, fears, resource scarcities and habit characteristics. Then, answer three questions listed below.

- Did you win the golden point and read Step 7 (Love it or leave it)?
- Do you have three points in more than a single category?
- Is the number of your negativity points above eight?

A positive answer is usually not a good sign, but for the first question it might be more complicated. If you've already resolved problems that led you to Step 7, you no longer need to worry. Otherwise, please multiply your negativity score by 1.5 before comparing with the threshold presented in the third question.

On the other hand, positive answer to the last two questions is a warning bell. Usually, you don't want to create such a negative change in your life. Therefore, please leave the current habit, unless your positive assessment gives you a highly desirable outcome (you will check it by calculating the positive score in the next section of this step).

You might be tempted to work on improving your negativity score. Please, do not do it now. Seriously! It could only harm you in the future. Instead, start by improving the positivity score to pass the threshold shown below.

Positivity score

Analyzing the positivity assessment's results is not a matter of numbers exclusively. Besides performing the calculation, you should also examine your feelings, intuition, and above all, the position of the habit in the need/want matrix.

The general threshold to pass in order to proceed with your habit contains three conditions:

- Your positivity score needs to be above eight points.
- Your habit of choice has to be present within the optimal need/want quadrant.
- You should genuinely feel that working on the particular habit is right in this exact moment of your life.

***

In order to establish the initial position of a chosen habit inside the need/want matrix, use your positivity results from the assessment. On the horizontal (need) line, mark your *need score* determined as the sum of points gathered for straightforward benefits and the hidden benefits. On the vertical (want) line, mark your *want score* determined as the sum of fun and pleasure as well as motivators.

Notice that zero is not at the cross point of lines to avoid a mistake. Also, remember that the initial position of your habit usually will change without doing any work by simply following the calculations described below.

If what you chose is closely related to your childhood dreams, magnify by 1.5 your positivity scores of every category rated equal or below two points. If you are not sure what your childhood dreams are, please search the Internet for *The Last Lecture* video by Randy Pausch. In fact, it is so powerful that even if you remember your dreams, probably you should watch it anyway.

If you desire the habit despite all costs, add up to two points to the want result (motivators or fun and pleasure categories). You are also obligated to do everything not to waste such a motivation. Therefore, you have to create enough need around the habit to put it into the best quadrant.

Similarly to an immense desire, there might exist a vast need. When the habit you want to establish is closely related to a deep need placed in one of the widest gaps on your personal pyramid of needs (go back to Step 4 for a refresher about that), add up to two points to your need score (straightforward and hidden benefits categories). Then, work as hard as you can to create more want if needed.

Another modifier of the positivity score is connected with your natural predispositions. If the habit uses your strengths and doesn't touch your weaknesses, please magnify the want score roots (fun and pleasure and motivators) by 1.5 for every result equal to or below two points.

***

When your habit passes the positivity threshold, it is definitely worth at least a serious trial to optimize and establish. On the other hand, if your case is not that clear, you have to give up your journey or bend the rules. The last option should not be overused, but sometimes it is decent. Such a case is valid when you failed to pass the threshold for your positivity assessment only marginally, or when you are certain that you could easily improve your positivity score during the optimization phase.

Please use your intuition and intellect to confirm whether you really want to slightly bend the rules. Also, keep in mind that if you cannot say an excited *yeah* to the challenge, you probably should say plain *no*.

Decision time

Once you have the results neatly calculated, it is time to make a decision to either follow or abandon the process of forming your habit of choice. The easiest situation occurs when positivity and negativity scores are on the proper side of the respective thresholds. In such an ideal case, definitely go through all steps, and then establish the routine.

On the other hand, when you have only positive score under control, you should at least go through the optimization stage. Usually in such a situation, you will be able to improve your scores enough to ensure success with a chosen habit formation.

When you have negativity and positivity scores below expectations, forget the habit and move on to the next one. However, the final decision is again up to you. After all, it is your life, and you are responsible for successes and failures. Therefore, use your instinct and logic to make the right decision considering your current situation. Add some modifiers or another category to the assessment if it feels appropriate. Remember you are unique. Thus, the system that serves you best should be individualized. Do what you must and decide cleverly.

If you have chosen to leave the habit, please try with another one. If you have decided to proceed, let's move on to the next step.

Tasks:

- Note the sum of all negativity points as the initial negativity score.
- Answer the questions and modify the negativity score as requested.
- Calculate the initial scores for need and want, and check the habit's position in the need/want matrix.
- Answer the modification questions presented in this chapter and modify the score accordingly.
- Compare scores with the thresholds and decide to either give up or follow the process of the chosen habit formation.

Step 9
The 0.7 version of your approach

In order to proceed to the optimization step, you need to make a draft for your work. Writing a rough outline of your approach to establish the chosen habit is the best way to generate the momentum of optimization. It might seem like a waste of time, but it has tremendous value.

You have probably never wondered how exactly writers write a book. Until I started writing this one, I didn't know either. Then I learned that almost every book begins its life as a rough draft. The purpose of the first phase of manuscript creation is to finish the whole thing as fast as possible. The result is usually extremely crappy, but no one cares, as the unpolished version will never be published. However, it is a necessary step of publication.

The rough draft is optimized during the process called editing. First, a manuscript is edited for content. After that, it is edited for style, often multiple times. Then in the final round, the book is proofread for typos and other mistakes, mostly grammatical ones.

After all the editorial steps, the book on the shelf is very different from the first sub-par version of the manuscript. People in the outside world see only the outcome, so they are often unaware of everything that came before. You might have been such a person just a minute ago. But now you can clearly see that book could never hit stores without being a crappy manuscript at the beginning.

Why am I talking about the editorial process? Because you will adapt the same principle to plan your habit launch.

Please open the workbook and create a rough draft of your plan to succeed. Feel free to use all the information gained during the positivity and negativity assessments. Remember that done is better than perfect. At this stage, you should make a plan that reflects the problems identified within the previous steps. Do not fix anything yet! Do not worry about optimization; you will improve the plan in the next step. In fact, some apparent mistakes are even desirable, as their existence will allow you to make small, easy and obvious changes to generate the momentum of success right from the beginning of the optimization process.

When you finish making a rough draft, move to the next step, which is all about the improvement of your 0.7 plan.

Tasks:

- Make a rough draft of your plan of formation of a chosen habit.

Step 10
Moving to 1.0 version of your plan

The process of optimization is all about answering one question:

How could the habit establishment process be changed to provide more of what you want and need and less of the negative side effects?

In other words, you should seek opportunities to increase the value and decrease the cost of the habit. This is the first (and the only one you need to know) law of a beneficial habit economy.

***

According to the Newton's law of dynamics, breaking the inertia at the starting point requires the most force. After the initial struggle, the momentum is much easier to maintain. Use this law to your advantage, warm up your mental muscles, and get your mind into a working state.

Look at your rough plan. Are there any obvious, general changes you could make right away? Without hesitation, write down such apparent improvements to start the ball rolling.

***

After the warm-up, use the impetus to move straight to the most painful parts of the plan. Do not elaborate on this task, as your brain already knows what is crucial to improve or eliminate. Do not overthink, and take only sixty seconds to write down the critical obstacles to deal with.

Then, ask how you can change the situation. This is the time for drastic changes, so do not restrict yourself or compromise over your long-term well-being. If you want to craft a completely new routine to get similar benefits, do it now. Consider creating a major goal related to your chosen habit. Make other huge changes if needed, as this stage is the last opportunity to think big efficiently. Therefore, go to the broadest perspective you can imagine and act bravely. I'm a very logical man, but I have to stress that during this phase you should also listen to your feelings and intuition.

***

After incorporating the biggest and the most emotional changes, comes time for methodical, logical work. Now, when you have huge issues resolved, you might be tempted to skip the rest of the optimization stage. Such a temptation derives from the belief that tiny improvements are less valid and somewhat unimportant; the belief that is very common, but also very wrong.

Tiny changes do matter. Making small improvements is the easiest path to create a huge difference. Because each mini-step in the right direction is worth many huge steps taken randomly, little things add up much quicker than most of us realize. Therefore, take the first step no matter how insignificant it looks. Then take another one. Continue this seemingly slow movement and sooner than you could have ever dreamed, you will achieve massive results.

I know it sounds like some sort of a mystical trash-talk. But this is the same process that made Toyota the biggest car manufacturer in the world. It is known under many names, but the core aspects are based on the Japanese's Kaizen philosophy of the compound effect of tiny improvements.

It is a powerful strategy, so never underestimate it. Instead, absorb the importance of the Kaizen philosophy in the light of habit formation by doing a little exercise.

Imagine that your road to success is a trail to the top of a mountain. Then visualize multiple rocks on this uphill road. Make this image vivid in your mind.

Tiny obstacles you're going to remove during optimization are such small rocks that, if left in their places, could create a serious issue. A single small rock is not a problem, but when you leave many, they could snowball into an avalanche and bury your path to success.

Let me guess that you do not want to let your dream die like that. Especially, when you can easily prevent it from happening. Do not hesitate. Remove the rocks one by one and with them the risk of a catastrophe. Approach every little improvement as a lifesaving effort, and you will no longer suffer from lack of motivation to take small steps.

***

After recognizing the usefulness of the Kaizen approach, optimize your plan with attention to details. Remember to deal not only with positive, but also with negative aspects of your habit of choice. Below you will find a brief description of actions related to those two areas.

1. When you work on minimizing negativity, you should concentrate your effort on *elimination* and *substitution*. Additionally, move away from your *weaknesses* whenever possible. The goal is to preserve all the positivity while reducing what could harm you.

2. Working on maximizing the positive features is about creating more *fun, excitement* and *benefits*. Additionally, you should look for creative ways to incorporate your inner *strengths* into the process.

Summarizing, working on optimization is simply

answering the question you already know. Here it is again:

How could the habit establishment process be changed to provide more of what you want and need and less of the negative side effects?

It is a powerful question, but it may feel too generic for most people. Therefore, let me show you how to be more specific in your efforts. Below you will find a list of the most common actions to consider when improving the formation of your chosen habit. They are presented as questions and categorized for clarity. Reading them is a good place to start, but do not stop there as those questions are only examples.

Following them blindly will lead you only to mediocre success. If you want to create something better, you will need to individualize the list. You are unique, so no one else can spot proper places for improvements. Thus, it is you who must personalize entries to reflect your exact situation.

There is a place in the workbook to note such ideas. Please do it while reading, but do not take any breaks. Seriously, do not stop until you have nothing left in your mind. Trust me on this, and you will finish the whole process at least two times faster. Make the list as long as you want, but do all the work in a single session. Otherwise, you will procrastinate and get subpar results.

Also, remember that the optimization process is often nonlinear. Therefore, do not hesitate to go back to already-passed points when needed, and add more notes whenever you feel an impulse to do so.

***

After creating the list of questions, you have to answer them all. Then, use the answers to improve your habit establishment plan. The whole process is easier to show than to describe, so look below for the sample questions, answers and suggestions. Use this incomplete starting list as a guide to make your own optimization efforts.

The common optimization categories

First, let me show you the table of contents for this part of the chapter.

1. Positivity increase
a) Motivation
b) Benefits
c) Fun
d) Your own ideas
2. Making it easier
a) Saving resources
b) Mindset first
c) Preparation
d) Your own ideas
3. Negativity limitation/inhibition
a) Negative habits
b) Negative emotions
c) Your own ideas

Quickly scanning over the outline reveals three key areas to concentrate on during your optimization process and several subcategories designed for your own ideas.

You are the one who possesses the fullest knowledge of your situation. Thus, you are the most qualified person to fill in those blank spaces. My job is just to encourage you; your job is to improve your plan by utilizing all the information, acquired by reading this book. Therefore, feel free to reread previous chapters for more sparks of inspiration, and remember to refer to previous notes when needed. And above all, put into your optimization some real effort.

The previous parts of this book prepare you well to go through descriptions of categories. While reading them, remember your job and make sure you have the workbook and all notes at hand. If you're ready, let's dig in.

***

1. Positivity increase

The core question here is: *How to increase the want and need components of the chosen habit?* Look at common subcategories below; then explore the related potential for improvement.

a) Motivation

The classic motivation tactic is the carrot and stick approach. Based on behavioral studies, the positive reinforcement usually gives stronger and more consistent effects, but statistics are correct for a population, not an individual, so always verify what works for you. Then, ask: *How could I include rewards and/or punishments in my plan?*

Answer the question using information from Chapter 6 and suggestions presented below.

Incorporate into your plan prizes to give yourself after achieving victories, but ensure to reward only true milestones. For example, when I was writing this book, I celebrated each finished rough draft of a chapter, and later, every finished revision of a full manuscript.

You too should reward yourself only for substantial results. Optimally, give yourself a bite of a personal carrot less often than every five repetitions completed. For your own good, use the external reward (not directly related to habit outcomes) not as the main force driving you to establish a habit, but only as a tool to generate momentum.

***

Another standard source of motivation is accountability. Yet, from the untrained perspective, some scientific papers show that accountability helps, while others make the opposite statement. How is that possible?

There are simply various forms of accountability. Therefore, do not question whether accountability could improve your chance of success. Instead, ask: *What type of accountability do I need to achieve outstanding results?* The answer depends on personal predispositions and preferences.

If you are similar to me, all the accountability you need is accountability to yourself. In such a case, for the best results, write a habit journal. Take a notebook or calendar and mark days when you succeed and days when you fail regarding your chosen habit.

Do not worry about little failures. Give yourself a 10-15% (but no more) margin for fiascos, as such a percentage of disasters would not interfere with your habit formation. When mini-failure happens, just note it in your journal/calendar. Then, forget about the issue and concentrate again on success. Remember that as long as you do not quit, your failure is only temporary. You might be defeated in a single battle, but there is still a war to win.

In your journal, you might note additional information for analysis of the habit establishment progress. It is completely supplementary, but sometimes worth the effort. For example, writing down the circumstances of slip-ups often helps in finding the reason behind the failures and, in consequence, eliminating or minimizing them. However, you must decide alone how much info you want to collect.

***

Many people are not solo warriors and could greatly improve their success rate by utilizing accountability to others. The most common way to do this is to find a partner who will ask you regularly (maybe even daily) about your progress with the habit formation.

You might also benefit from finding a person who will take on a similar challenge. There are communities for aspiring runners, writers and even early-risers. You can easily find one related to your particular challenge on Facebook or by searching with Google. Do it if it feels suitable.

You are the only one able to say whether to tell your friends, family or others in your community about your mission. You could even state it publicly to the whole world. However, before making the decision, think whether your challenge will interfere with the lives of others.

For example, if it will influence the lives of your family members, you have to tell them. Additionally, consider asking your relatives for encouragement. Often explaining to them how important the habit is to you is enough. They love you and want you to flourish, so do not disappoint them with a mediocre effort.

b) Benefits

You should always seek opportunities to add additional benefits, both obvious and hidden, to your habit. Therefore, during optimization stage, ask: *How can*

I include more benefits?

The answer varies from one person to another. My only suggestion is not to restrict yourself, and to stretch your imagination. For example, if your habit is running, you might add benefits like:

- hanging with a friend
- listening to audiobooks
- reviving your mindset by affirmations and visualizations
- using the run as an opportunity to practice gratitude
- practicing some form of meditation
- using the time to reflect on various subjects
- using running as an excuse to connect with nature
- seeing the sunset from a more suitable place
- passing a beautiful neighbor, every morning
- and whatever else feels like a benefit to you

c) Fun

The question to ask here is: *How can I add additional fun, pleasure, gamification, etc. to the habit of choice?*

The answer might be as trivial as creating some kind of a competition. Ask your friends for participation or create a public online challenge to get the ball rolling.

Some people like to treat their trial as an experiment. I'm one of those science geeks who find pleasure in measurements, systematic observation and analysis. Maybe you are similar. Or maybe you find pleasure and fun in something else. The possibilities for adding fun are personal and always in abundance.

You probably will not guess what type of optimization gave me the most fun when I was forming my running habit. But you do not have to wonder, as I will gladly tell you my little dirty secret.

I just loved the confused faces of the people I passed by. They could not believe what they had just seen. However, I can't blame them. After all, you do not often see a smiling, barefoot guy running on the pavement. What does this tell us about fun? If something as trivial as taking off my shoes created so much fun and pleasure for me, nothing is too small or too strange to give similar results to you.

***

Although our predispositions regarding fun and pleasure greatly vary, there is one generic powerful technique to boost fun and motivation. In fact, it is so mighty that you should consider staying away from it to ensure you will not suffer from possible side effects.

I hope you are now intensely wondering what the heck this deadly weapon is. Let me pause (of course for my fun and pleasure) and after that . . . relieve the tension.

It is a bet. It might look simple, but betting is a complex issue. It brings gamification to your plan. It is fun. It creates negative motivation in the form of fear of defeat; and it generates positive motivation in the shape of winning the stake of a bet. Betting is such a great technique that at first glance, it looks like the king of all tricks. But there is a reason why I have not mentioned it previously.

Betting has its dark side. It is dangerous and highly addictive. If you are a typical gambler, do yourself a favor and never bet. In such a case, you have to cure, not reinforce your gambling addiction, as it is usually not about the game itself, but about the failures. That is why gambling addicts stop playing only after a loss and never after a win. You do not want to create addiction to failure, do you? So use betting sparingly and always with full awareness of the pros and cons of the technique.

d) Your own ideas

Add to the list anything that feels right. You can include supplementary categories, subcategories or particular questions at any point. Remember that even the smallest improvement counts, as nothing is too trivial if it works for you. Therefore, be bold and optimize the plan as much as you can.

2. Making it easier

The core question here is: *How can I make the formation of the chosen habit easier?*

People often quit because they needlessly try to do the job the hard way. Sometimes it is pure stubbornness; more often, it is just a lack of knowledge. But wisdom is learnable.

For around three thousand years, sage men have been saying we should be like water. Water always looks for the easiest way to flow, yet it always flows to its target. It moves around obstacles, and when it cannot, it uses persistent force to break through obstructions over the long run.

Look at the Grand Canyon, one of the incredible accomplishments of water, and admire the power of the flexible approach. The Colorado River meanders to find the easiest route, but at the same time, almost effortlessly shapes the rock with persistent action. Therefore, I repeat after Bruce Lee, "Be water, my friend."

Open your mind, use your imagination, and look for opportunities to make your journey easier. But also acknowledge that sometimes you might need to make a persistent effort to crush an obstacle. Be as flexible as you can and find a balanced (easy, but bulletproof) way to establish the chosen habit and improve your life.

Notice that while persistence alone could lead you to amazing results, I recommend using it only as a last resort. Unless you love avoidable work, always begin with making your habit formation easier, starting from suggestions described below.

a) Saving Resources

The first question you should ask to make the process of habit establishment easier is: *How could I save resources?*

The simplest answer hides in a problem-solving principle called Occam's razor, and in a pharmacological concept of the Minimum Effective Dose. Both rules are combined and compactly articulated in a quotation commonly ascribed to Albert Einstein – *"Everything should be made as simple as possible, but not simpler."*

In such a light, all you need to create a habit is a tiny effort. However, you have to make that effort every single day. Consistency is the essence of routine formation. Even a small action performed daily will allow you to form a beneficial habit. Therefore, ask yourself: *Could I start with a smaller step?*

Why waste time when you can achieve your main goal and establish a habit with a minimal effective investment smaller than five minutes daily? Of course, you can scale up later, but only if you successfully form a habit firstly.

***

Apply the minimalist philosophy concerning equipment and other investments. Save your money, time, willpower and other resources. At the beginning, you should spend your assets almost exclusively on performing the minimal amount of the core part of activity regularly. Borrow stuff instead of buying. Look for cheaper alternatives or use your imagination and find what you need for free. More money put in does not always return a better outcome. Many people do dips on their kitchen chairs with impressive results.

***

Of course, not every type of resource spending is equal. You have to decide how much money, time, willpower and energy you want to invest to create favorable circumstances for your chosen habit formation. Nevertheless, I would like to stress a useful, but rarely exploited way to use resources.

Apart from putting in minimal effort consistently, consider trading one resource for another. For example, you could spend money to save willpower, time and energy.

Some people hire a personal fitness instructor who shouts at them. The primary role of such a trainer is not what you usually think. The most important benefit of hiring a personal coach is to save willpower. He remembers to come regularly so you do not have to. He screams at you so you save willpower you would normally use to motivate yourself. He also provides you curated instructions so you save time and energy that you otherwise would have to spend on learning.

Spending to preserve other resources might be a great investment. Not to mention that mastering such trading is simpler than playing in the stock market. Just ask what resource is the most important for your habit formation.

Then, look for the possibilities to trade abundant resources for the crucial one you lack.

***

Summarizing this subcategory, I want to repeat: *Start slowly*. I know that some people say that to ensure willpower and self-discipline you must achieve notable success as fast as possible. I have to admit it is true, but only partially. Even the biggest success is not enough to make you happier if it's not in alignment with your core values and creates too much tension in your life. Unfortunately, the latter is a common beginner's mistake.

Professionals always look for the fields congruent with their personal advantages. Many pro athletes begin as soccer players but then go for basketball because of their growth. Other sportsmen start as cyclists but switch to triathlons after a while. Steven Pressfield began his writing career writing ads, then he wrote screenplays, and finally he found his purpose in writing books. If you want to succeed, learn from such people, do not play against the odds, act like a pro, and avoid amateurish mistakes.

Think more about pro athletes. Do they start from the highest level? Of course they do not, as it is the guaranteed way to serious injuries. Instead, they start slowly, build a base, and then aim for peak performance. Moreover, they utilize the similar approach every single season.

If you want to succeed with habits, try to mimic the approach of pro sportsmen. Pick the right discipline, start slowly and build your routine gradually. Otherwise, you will end like many young talents who were expected to become great but never fulfilled those hopes because of injuries. Do not copy their mistakes, and always have a long-term game plan in the back of your head.

***

Techniques described above are just the tip of the iceberg. Nevertheless, they should be enough to inspire you to find other ways to save resources needed for habit establishment and an energized life. For best results, analyze your particular situation, be creative, and optimize what you can remembering about personal advantages.

b) Mindset first

Thousands of books teach how to improve mindset to increase outcomes you get from life actions. So many books are written on the subject for a reason. According to numerous scientific studies, your attitude influences the probability of your success.

Therefore, during the optimization of a habit formation plan, ask: *How could I boost my self-confidence and create a better mindset for beneficial routines and a better life?*

In fact, the above question might be the foremost one to answer. A strong, negative mindset can ruin your entire effort to establish a habit, as you need at least a moderately positive attitude to improve the quality of your life.

But for some people, it is difficult to admit. A few years ago, I too thought that all this hype about the importance of mindset was bullshit. In fact, I still don't believe in a majority of psychological fluff, and recommend such an approach to you.

Part of the reason behind that is lack of transparency in psychology compared with stricter sciences. As you see in various books, magazines and scientific journals, results of psychological studies often lead to opposite conclusions. Moreover, if something works for six out of ten people, journalists and authors tend to treat it is as a universal rule. Sometimes, I'm really sick of it. But mindset is a different cup of tea as it can easily pass a logical verification.

Even if you are a rationality maniac (like me most of the time), you have already observed the power of mindset. You have witnessed the effectiveness of brainwashing by sects, armies, corporations, television, etc. Undoubtedly, you have seen people who developed such different mindsets that you could not believe they were the same persons you had known before.

Acknowledge that attitude is changeable and hugely influences your life. Only after that can you enhance your mindset to serve you. Usually, seeing the importance of a subject is all it takes to improve your attitude enough for the purpose of this book.

Of course, if you want, you could mimic the techniques used for brainwashing, for your good not evil. However, you do not have to be such an extremist. Often, buying a solid mindset creation book allows you to begin your self-development.

Start this journey by accepting that you absolutely need at least a slightly positive mindset to successfully improve your existence by implementing beneficial habits in various areas of your life. This is especially crucial if you are overly pessimistic or have a low self-esteem. Honing such a negative mindset is like asking for a failure.

In such a case, buy a good book and establish the mindset-related habits, starting from the easiest and most productive ones like: practicing smiling, gratitude journaling, objective analysis of limiting beliefs, cultivation of a slightly positive attitude, visualizations, affirmations, getting small things done, etc. Be consistent, do not judge the techniques before trying them, and then adopt only what works for you. After that, you will thank me for including this "fluffy" subcategory, unless you stubbornly take inaccurate actions.

For example, I constantly see people ditching the idea of the importance of mindset because of a common mistake regarding positive affirmations. Most people incorrectly concentrate on the outcomes while they should think about the process.

Thus, never say "I'm slim" when you are not. Instead, say something like "I perform the habit of exercising and healthful eating daily so I will be slim." At the same time, always visualize that you practice a chosen routine. Combining visualization with affirmations is widely used by many successful professionals, including Tiger Woods, Michael Masterson and Michael Jordan. Now you also know how to do this efficiently.

The above instruction is an excellent example of how important the proper groundwork is, even for something that looks easy and obvious at the first glance (like visualizations, affirmations or formation of a habit). Speaking of accurate preparation, let's move on to the next subcategory.

c) Preparation

Preparation is essential if you are serious about any type of a desired outcome. The question to ask here is: *What can I do in advance to make habit creation easier?*

Reflecting on the above question, notice that you have answered it multiple times. Each finished exercise from this book is such an answer. Your work put into optimization is a preparation.

However, what you have done already could not be the only preparation you want to secure. For example, you might want more information about your habit of choice. Some knowledge is indeed necessary, but be aware of the paralysis of analysis syndrome.

To ensure that you will not use insufficient knowledge as an excuse, define beforehand what is sufficient to start. Do not try to learn everything at the beginning. Instead, gather only *enough high-quality information* for the first week of routine practice.

***

Another example of preparation is scheduling the starting point of your routine. Usually the best time to start is soon after writing your optimized plan. Waiting up to three days is optimal in most cases.

However, sometimes you should postpone the habit creation. For example, if you want to establish a jogging routine, winter is probably not the ideal time to start. Bad weather will drain your energy and willpower to go out and run. Therefore, you should consider scheduling the starting point in a more favorable season. After deciding on the exact date, mark it on your calendar and relentlessly stick to it.

Always choose the most advantageous moment for starting your beneficial habit formation. This rule applies to the season of the year as well as the hour of the day. Technically most habits can be practiced at any time, but this doesn't mean you should put them randomly into your agenda. Instead, schedule your new habit in the best possible time to benefit your life.

Another possibility is to do your habit in the morning.

There is more than one reason why books about morning routines are so common. Authors usually share only that such a routine schedule can pump you up for the rest of a day. But there is much more.

Think about your mornings. Most of the time, you are on autopilot, aren't you? This natural human tendency to automate morning activities can be used to your advantage. You can easily replace habits or incorporate new ones between two that are already established.

The third reason is the nature of willpower, which is strongest in the morning, as sleep refills this resource. Therefore, accessing willpower at the first part of the day is the easiest. For centuries, many renowned artists have known this, and have done most of their work before breakfast or anything else. You can mimic them for your own good. For example, if you have a severe willpower issue with habit creation, perform the routine as one of the first things in your day whenever possible.

***

Of course, the shown examples only scratched the surface. Most of the preparation has not even been touched. But you are the only one able to explore it entirely. So prepare as well as you can in a quick manner, and jump into action, as even the fullest preparation is useless if you don't make use of it.

3. Negativity limitation/inhibition

Dealing with this category, ask: *How can I eliminate, substitute or minimize the negativity related to my habit of choice?*

a) Negative habits

Other habits might negatively interfere with your chosen routine. In fact, this is a common issue, vastly overlooked by inexperienced habit makers.

Sometimes the already formed routines decrease the probability of creation of a new habit by driving you in the opposite direction. This is a problem, as when you try to forge a beneficial habit, you expect benefits. However, when at the same time you still practice bad routines, your results will depend not only on the habit of choice but also on your current lifestyle.

Please recall the figures from the Chapter 2 and the importance of going straight to the outcome. Then acknowledge that you cannot go in the opposite direction with different routines/activities and expect to arrive to the target.

For example, when you try to establish an exercise routine, and you expect one of the benefits to be weight loss, do not sabotage your effort with a habit of eating tons of sweets daily. Before you can concentrate on exercising, first cope with your bad habit. Otherwise, you will mask your bad habits with good ones. It might look like a decent strategy for an amateur, but it is like using deodorant instead of taking a shower. So just don't do it.

***

Some habits directly influence the effects of your habit of choice, others act indirectly. The latter ones are much more common so we have a natural tendency to ignore them. However, these tricky negative habits often substantially decrease the likelihood of forming a beneficial habit by robbing you of the resources you need. They steal your time, money, energy, etc. When you see a thief in your life, you stay away for a good reason.

Similarly, avoid the thieves of your precious life resources. Television and Internet consumption are the most widespread, but other routines can be equally harmful. Thus, minimize their influence, or better yet, remove them from your life.

***

You can look at the elimination of a bad habit from many angles. However, usually the best way to eradicate an undesirable routine is by replacing it with another activity. To perform such an operation as easy and fast as possible, you require knowledge about the classic three-step model of a habit. According to it, habits can be simplified to a three-step loop.

1. The first step is a cue or trigger to do the automatic activity. It might be a particular person, place, time, feeling, or anything else. For example, some people smoke when their colleagues do. Others take a cigarette as a supplement to drinking beer or every time they feel stressed. Some smoke after settling into a comfortable armchair, others smoke mostly in a bar or just after waking up. The possibilities are endless and very personal.

Fortunately, despite the nature of your trigger, the easiest way to reduce the negative influence of a bad habit is simple and generic. All you have to do to decrease the negative outcomes of a bad habit by 80% is to avoid the cues related to the particular routine. But often it is inconvenient. Additionally, 80% reduction is worse than complete elimination. Therefore, consider using a more complicated approach and substitute your bad habit with a better one as described later.

2. After the trigger, comes the second step, which is

the habitual activity itself. For the ambitious habit builder, it is an opportunity to put your own routine in the place of the bad habit. Yes, you could put a new habit under the existing triggers. It is not easy but doable. However, you need to choose the right routine to install, as it has to go through the same, or very similar, third step of the loop.

3. The last step of the habit is a reward. While you might imagine it as something materialistic, usually it is more elusive. Often the reward is hard to recognize at first glance and may be easily overlooked, because you learnt to ignore the habitual feeling of satisfaction you get from the already-established routines (either bad or good). However, the lack of awareness does not make striving for the reward less relevant. Instead, your subliminal drive to achieve such emotional prizes is often very strong.

The feeling you mindlessly look for might be: stress removal, a slight decrease of anxiety, an increase of belonging and acceptance, a spark of love, better mood, some happiness, an accomplishment, or almost anything else that you crave.

Moreover, rewards you expect to gain from various routines are often the opposite. Sometimes you search for something that energizes you while in other cases for relaxation. This means that during the analysis of a reward, you must ignore (for a moment) your general preferences in life, and identify the specific prize linked to the particular trigger and routine.

****

If you want to replace a bad habit with a new, good one, you need to recognize the trigger and the reward. In order to do so, apply some mindfulness into your daily actions around the negative habit.

When you catch yourself on performing a bad routine, ask yourself what pushed you to do that. It is that easy to recognize your cue. Moreover, this trigger is often a reflection of the reward. When the cue is a stressful situation, the obvious reward you seek is stress relief. When the trigger is in the form of a particular person, the reward is often socialization and acceptance.

You might wonder why so few people perform this analysis if it's so easy. It's simply due to the nature of habitual routines, as you perform them on autopilot, mindlessly, without consciously elaborating on them.

Fortunately, with just a tiny effort, you can act slightly less automatically and turn your mind on for a moment to analyze the trigger and reward of the bad habit you would like to substitute. After that, replace the harmful action with a beneficial one. Of course, sometimes this is trickier than it sounds, but discussing dealing with possible difficulties is far beyond the scope of this book. Let me assume that those of you especially interested in this subject will find the proper advice in books targeting specific bad routines.

***

Summarizing this subcategory, the standard question to ask here is: *How could I minimize the effects of bad habits that I currently hone?* The more advanced question is: *How could I use my bad habits to create new beneficial routines utilizing triggers and rewards that already exist?*

b) Negative emotions

The question to ask here is: *How can I eliminate or minimalize what creates negative emotions about the chosen habit?*

The answer usually utilizes some form of fixing the reasons for hating particular aspects of a chosen habit formation. As you read in Chapter 3, such causes could be either direct or indirect and are quite frequent. In that chapter, I also wrote that you would know what to do with those issues at the right time. Now, you are ready.

Acknowledge that most of the improvements from previous categories or subcategories indirectly limit the negative feelings in various ways. In fact, the still unaddressed emotional issues are rare. But sometimes they occur.

When it happens, go back to Chapter 3 for a refresher, look at your notes from previous exercises, and use all your powers to create custom-tailored questions to optimize your habit formation plan regarding negative emotions.

***

That was the last subcategory of the outline. However, as I have mentioned before, it is only a draft, an unfinished version to expand based on your personal taste and needs. Feel free to give your attention to other ways of optimizing your habit creation approach, as the presented list is incomplete even from my perspective.

Believe me, one could write a series of books on possible improvements to the habit creation process. However, often it is much faster and more effective to look deep inside your soul rather than reading endless volumes in search of a vague idea. Therefore, do some brainwork, improve all you can, and do not stop until you are happy with the result.

***

At the final stage of optimization, consider discussing your plan with someone else, as another pair of eyes can help you spot more opportunities. Personally, I recommend asking a spouse or close friend to provide feedback. Often such an editor proposes ways to improve your plan from a different point of view, prioritizing your relationship, which for most people, is part of their pyramid of needs anyway.

Remember that done is better than perfect, so do not aim for a flawless plan. Instead, spend a considerable amount of time and effort to create a plan, and then start moving in the right direction. You can always make improvements later, on the go, to maintain the correct course. However to be able to do so, you have to start somewhere.

I cannot stress enough how important it is to take action to make your theoretical plan a reality. Theory without practice will be a shameful waste of your time. After all, you do not want to create the habit of pointless procrastination, do you?

***

While this is a logical end of the chapter, I cannot finish without touching on complex habits. Therefore, if you were so stupidly brave to choose a complex habit to create, I have a reminder. Go back to Step 3 after analyzing a part of the chosen habit. As I have warned you, you will have to go through the whole process for all the sub-habits. Then, for the best possible outcome, compile all the results into one consistent, coherent approach.

Such thoughtful analysis is demanding to finish. Therefore, I want to mention a little shortcut that can give you 80% of the results for 20% of the difficulty. It will still be a challenge but a much more bearable one.

You can start the journey with the first sub-goal and

analyze the remaining sub-goals while already practicing the subroutine. You will sacrifice 20% of possible results due to the inconsistencies, but it might be an acceptable price to pay. Whichever path you decide to follow, stay positive and remember it is a long-term game.

***

While complex habits often need comprehensive preparation before starting the challenge, simple routines are less demanding. All you have to do after the optimization phase is go to the execution step with an open mind. By carrying out your approach mindfully, you will spot the opportunities for previously unseen improvements. It is completely normal, especially during the first week of the habit development. Do not waste those possibilities and optimize your beneficial habits as long as you can. In fact, the process is never finished as you are constantly changing, and so should your habits in order to reflect your actual situation.

Tasks:

- Optimize the rough draft by contemplating the question: How could the habit establishment process be changed to provide more of what you want and need and less of the negative side effects?
- Note obvious, generic changes you can make right away. Remember to refer to previous notes during the optimization.
- Identify the most painful parts of the plan.
- Take the widest perspective and think about drastic changes, as this is the last good stage to make them.
- Follow up with methodical, logical work on smaller improvements. Start by making a list of optimization

questions by picking from the examples.

- Using your feelings and intellect, add other questions that reflect your actual situation.
- Answer questions you've just noted. Optimize the positive and negative aspects of the habit of choice and create your optimized plan (sometimes multiple reiterations are needed).
- Optionally, if you have taken a complex habit, decide what to do after analysis of a habit, and do it.
- Read the final chapter of the book and execute your personalized habit establishment plan.
- Celebrate your successful habit launch . . . and repeat the process with a new habit.

THE GRAND FINALE

Take the optimal route and never give up

Whatever you plan to do, one of the best ways to simply improve your strategy is to intensify the positive emotional charge of the change. You cannot go wrong if you minimize bad emotions like anger, fear, etc., and simultaneously increase the amount of good emotions like faith, hope, and above all love.

However, even the best plan is worth nothing when you do not take action. So after you finish creating a plan for your optimal approach, you have to follow it. Like Richard Branson entitled one of his books, *Screw It, Let's Do It!*

Acknowledge that you have already done half of the hard work needed to succeed. Do not waste that effort. Repeat to yourself why you need and want the change. Maximize the fun, enjoy the process, and never give up.

I will not lie to you. No matter how exceptional your plan is, some obstacles will inevitably occur. A few of them may be even impossible to work around. This is how the world works, so just accept it. You cannot prepare for everything, and you should not try.

The aim of the optimization was not to prepare you for the unexpected. Instead, it was all about saving as much of your willpower, energy and self-discipline as possible. Remember that you have plenty of those resources, so giving up is not an option. Recognize that you preserved all these reserves to deal with random issues.

You may not feel it yet, but you will have everything you need to successfully defeat the majority of obstacles. Sometimes, you will use your creativity, and in other situations, you will utilize the brute-force approach. Be flexible, mimic what you have practiced earlier, and optimize steps during the journey, if needed.

Also, prepare for failures.

It is crucial to accept that you may fail in minor aspects like removing some stumbling blocks. But as long as you do not give up and follow the right route to the target, you will inevitably achieve at least 80% of the benefits from the habit you want to establish.

Moreover, this 80% will be worth much more than 100% of positive outcomes from the non-optimized 0.7 version of your approach. You would have to be crazy not to think that is a huge win, and I know that you are not insane. I also know that like a great strategist, you can be defeated in some battles and still win the war.

Speaking about war, it is not over until you either win or give up. As long as you persistently keep doing what needs to be done, your only option is to win. And the success will materialize sooner than you imagine . . .

Free PDF Workbook

Do exercises described in this book in a well-organized manner.

Bonus Material

Check out the bonus material for this book and get:

- Different points of views

- Extended information

- Additional examples

- And more

Get all the extras at:

http://moniuszko.net/habit-launch-extras/

I would like to thank you for purchasing and reading my book. I hope you liked reading it as much as I loved writing it. I know that if you follow the process you have learned, you will greatly improve your life. You will succeed with the habits you have previously failed to create (maybe even many times). When that happens, please let me know. Take a minute or two and share your opinion with the world.

Leave a review on Amazon or GoodReads and tell your friends how this book affected your life. I really will appreciate every single review, as I cannot stress enough the importance of feedback for self-publishing authors. Only with your help will I be able to continue to write books to positively change lives. Thank You!

After leaving a review, rinse and repeat what you've learned until you create all the routines that you want and need to thrive. Then shine as you were always meant to . . .

***

This book has been through many edits, but as English is not my native language, and nothing is infallible, you might catch a spelling error or other mistake. I would sure appreciate if you let me know when that happens to improve the future editions. You can contact me at moniuszko.grzegorz@gmail.com with the subject line "*Habit launch* mistake."

Acknowledgments

It would be impossible to thank everyone who has had an impact on the creation of this book. However, there are a few who deserve specific mention. I would like to especially thank:

- Michal Stawicki for his tremendous help with launching this book.
- My wife, Aleksandra and my mother, Danuta for their belief in my capabilities and their encouragement to never give up even when the journey becomes a little harder.
- My children, especially my son, Wojciech, who shows me every day that mindset can let you be happy despite any handicaps.
- My editor, Amanda. Her insights and suggestions made this book an immeasurably better read than the first, rough draft.
- Gosia Lewandowska for her encouragement and helping hand.
- The members of the Authority Self-Publishing Facebook Group.
- All the people who have shaped my thinking in any way . . .

About the Author

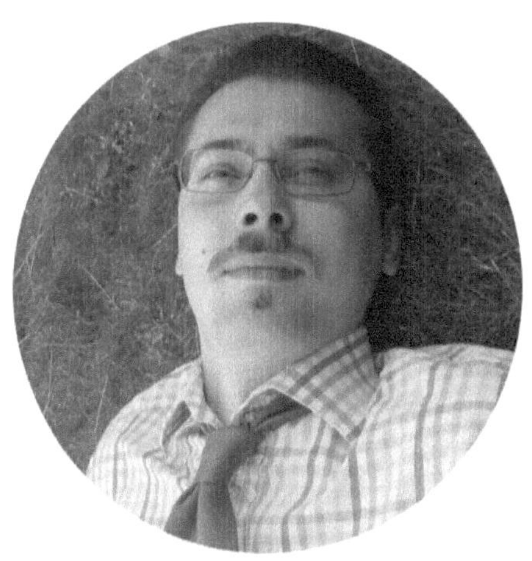

Gregor Moniuszko is an author, scientist, husband, father of two and a marathoner. Yet, whomever you ask would say the one adjective that best describes him is "lazy."

He writes books for people who have failed when trying to cope with simple, proven, detailed (you name it), methods. Usually, nonfiction books describe either general visions or detailed tips. But what readers need (and what Gregor provides) is a balanced mix of strategy and tactics with instruction on how to individualize them.

What separates Gregor from other authors is his respect for laziness and understanding of science (aka PhD). He also has a rare ability to share fresh and obvious ideas. Fresh, because they're overlooked. Obvious, in that they resonate with you so deeply you instantly know they are true.

Read more at Gregor's website at
http://moniuszko.net/about/

Notes

Notes

Notes

www.ingramcontent.com/pod-product-compliance
Lightning Source LLC
Chambersburg PA
CBHW031120250726

48655CB00004B/1772